Disclaimer
This coloring book is intended as a recreational and relaxation activity only.

It is not a medical or therapeutic product and should not be used as a substitute for professional diagnosis, treatment, or therapy of any kind.
The designs and accompanying information are created to provide enjoyment, promote calm, and encourage gentle creative engagement.

Every person's needs and abilities are unique. If you are caring for someone living with memory loss, Alzheimer's disease, or another cognitive condition, please follow the guidance of qualified healthcare professionals regarding appropriate activities and supervision.

The publisher and author are not responsible for any outcome resulting from the use or misuse of this book.

Always ensure a safe, comfortable environment while coloring, and use only non-toxic art materials suitable for the individual's abilities.

© Nevada Thornton - All rights reserved. No part of this book may be reproduced, distributed, or transmitted in any form or by any means without written permission from the publisher.

LARGE PRINT Coloring books
for adults relaxation

HAPPINESS

Thornton Nevada

Nature & Animals
(Gentle, relaxing, memory-evoking)

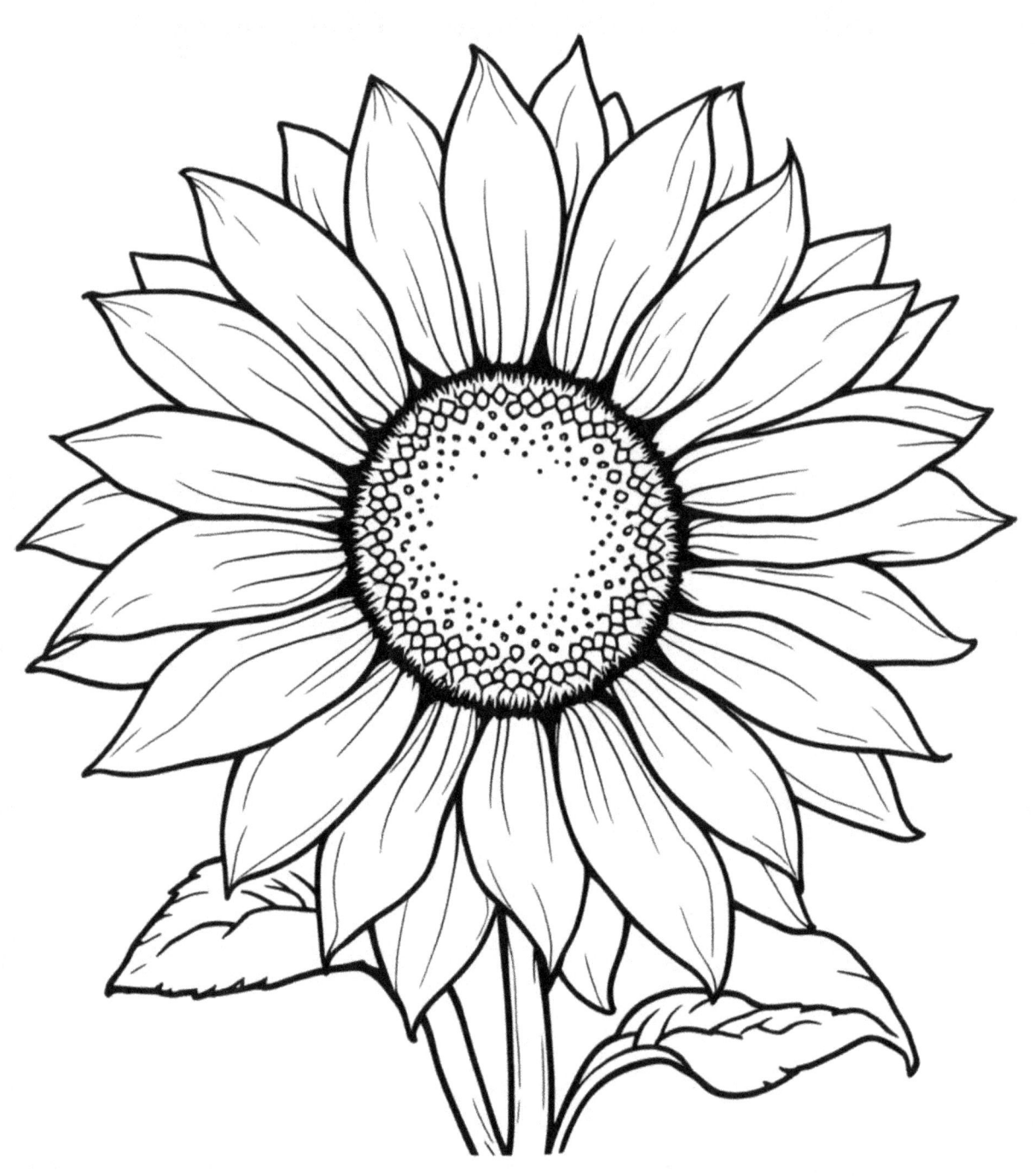

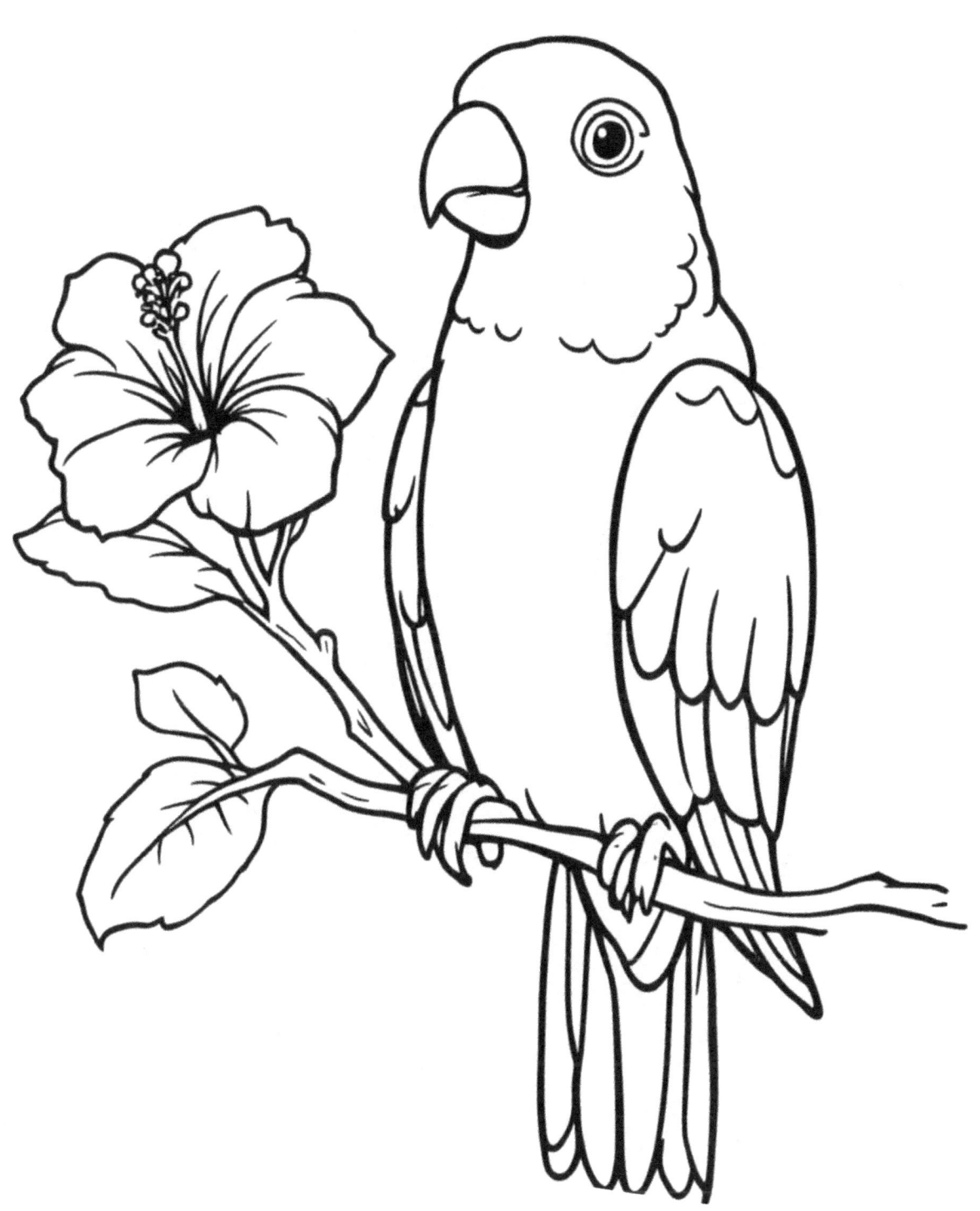

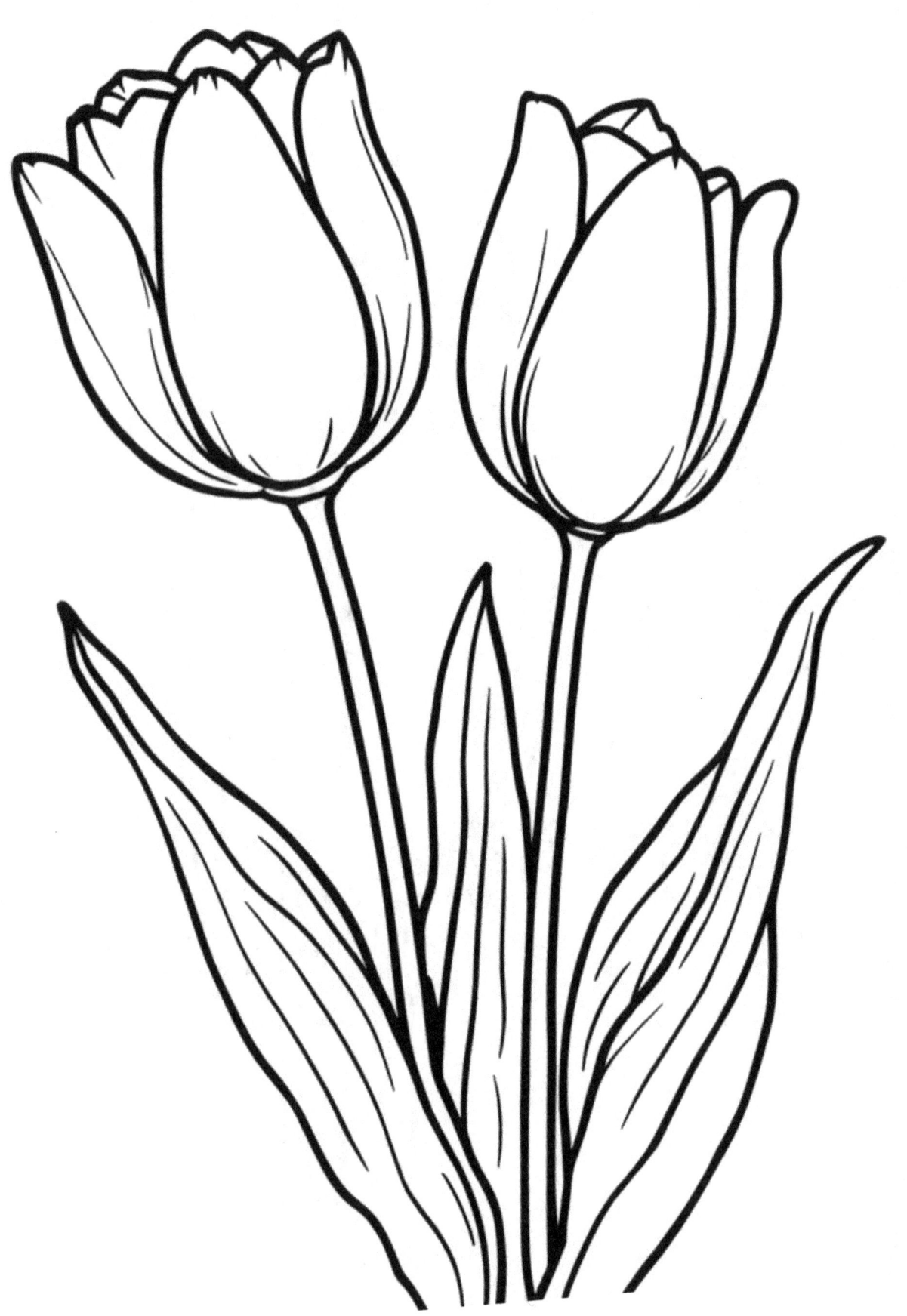

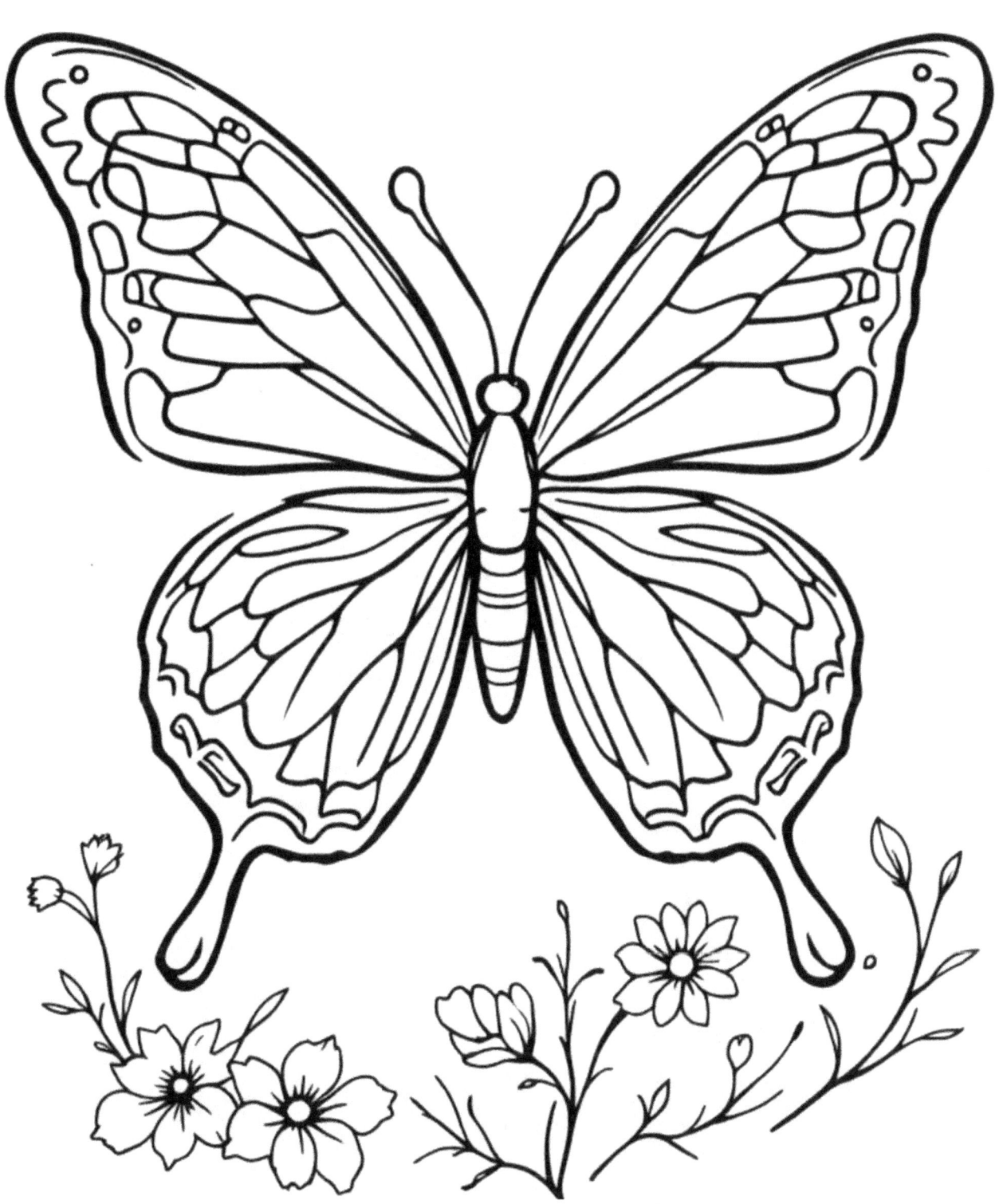

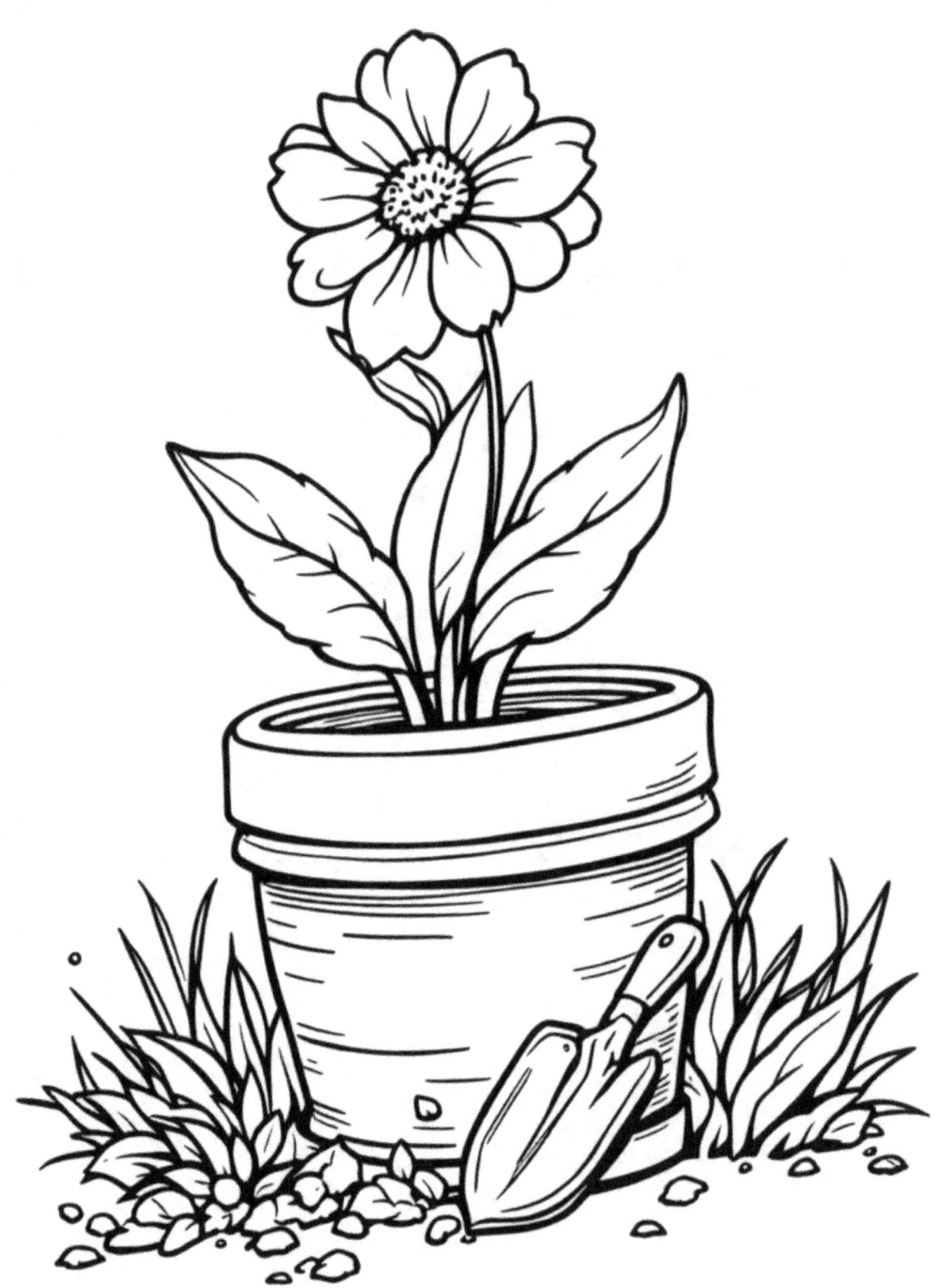

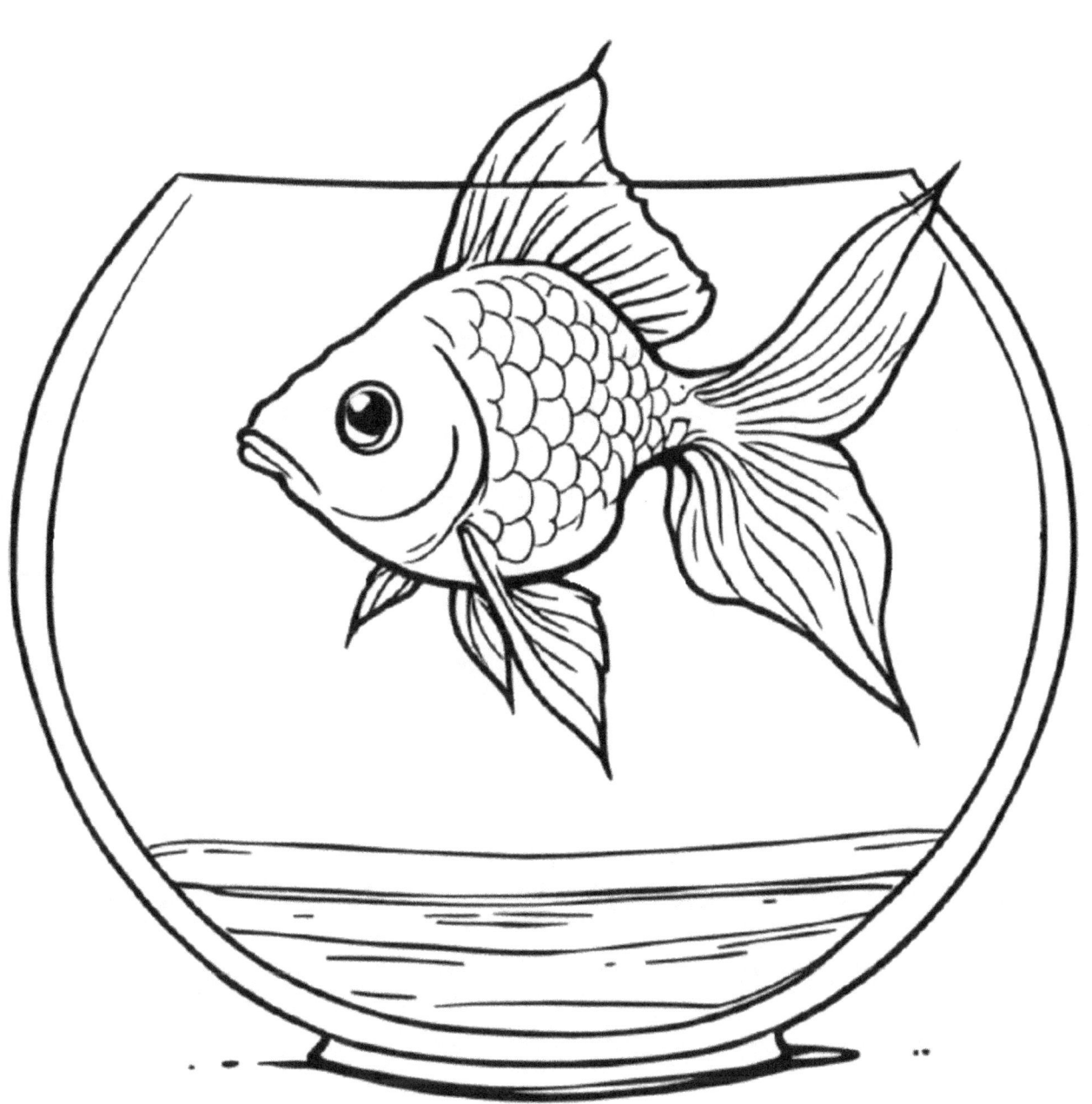

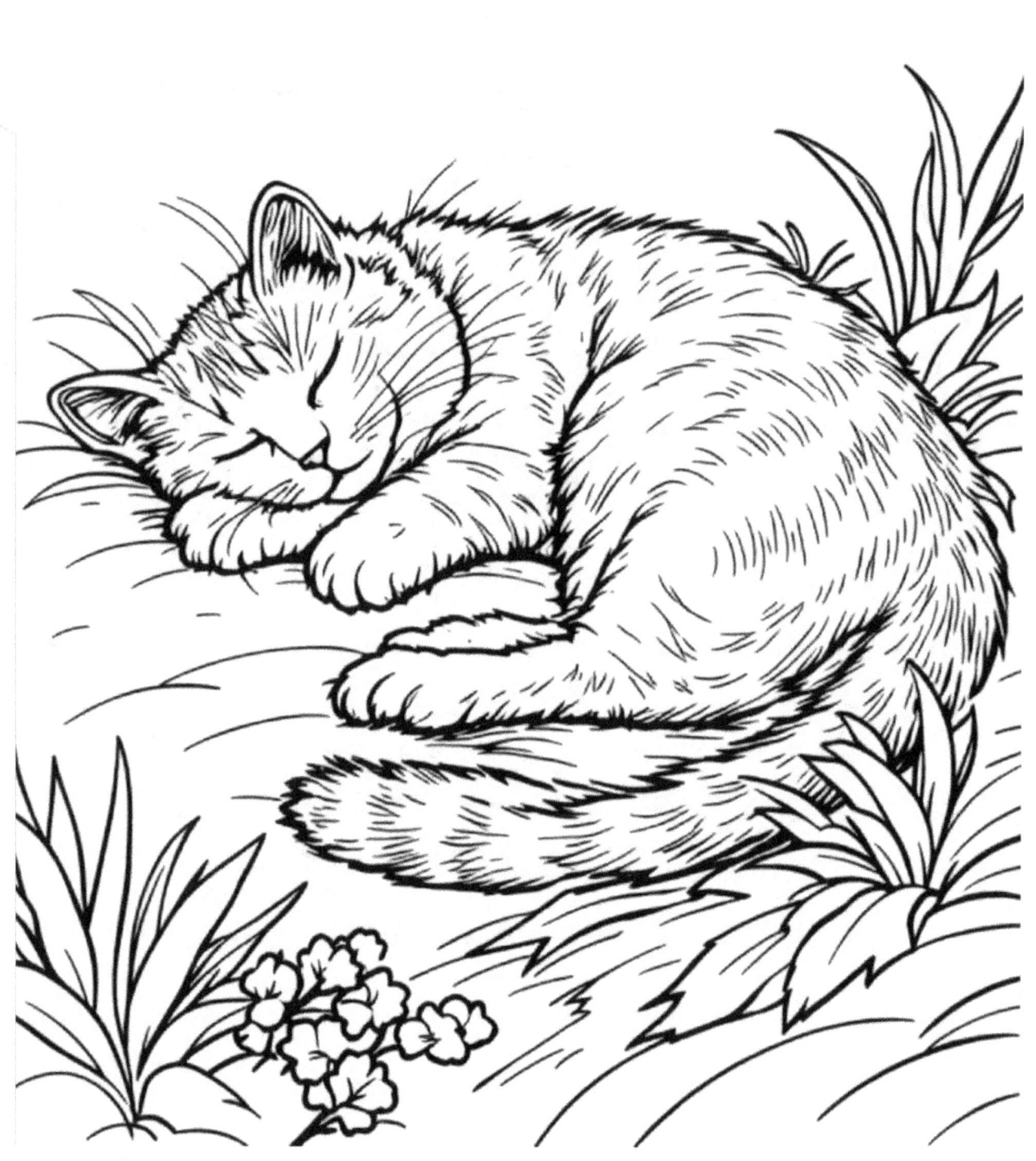

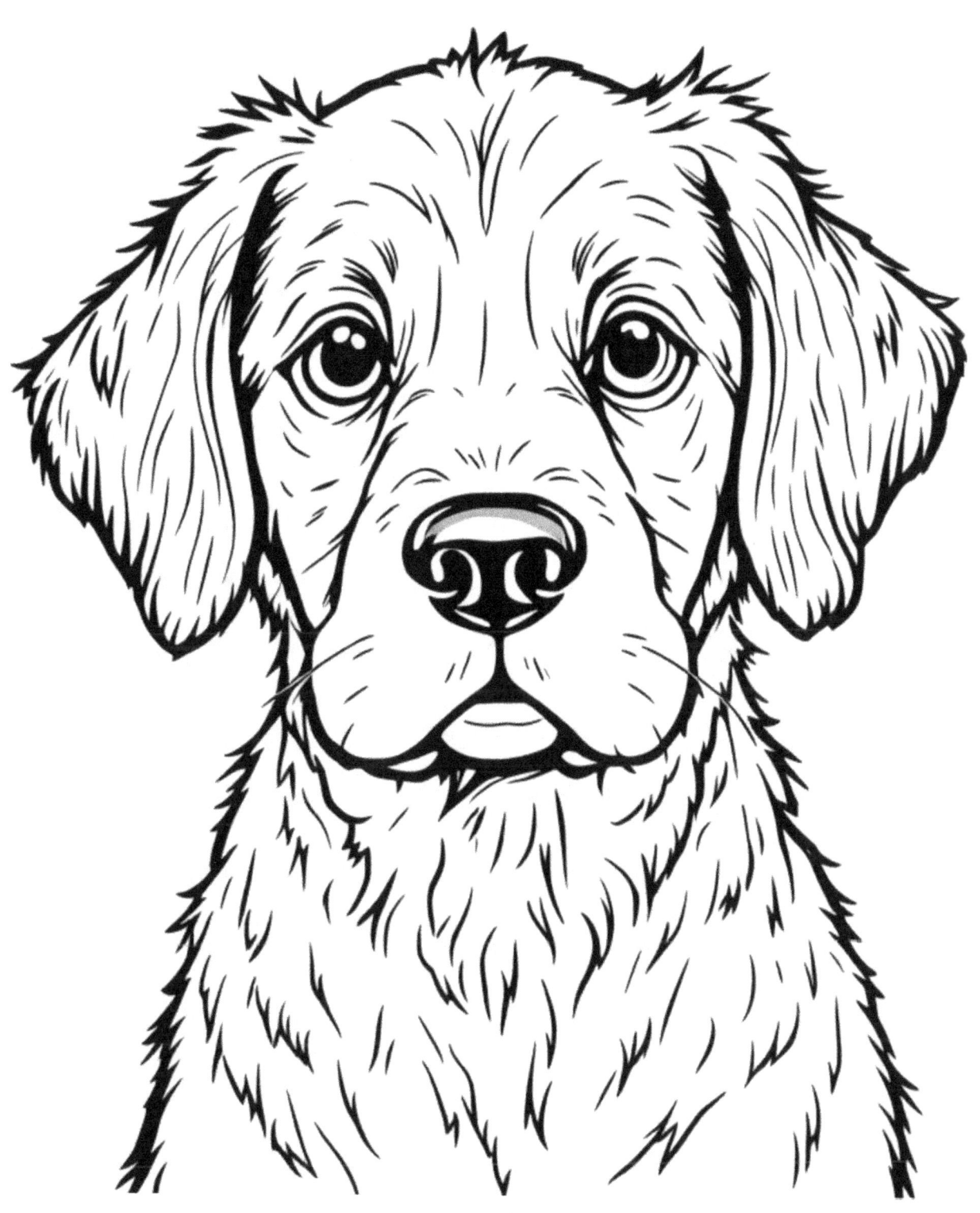

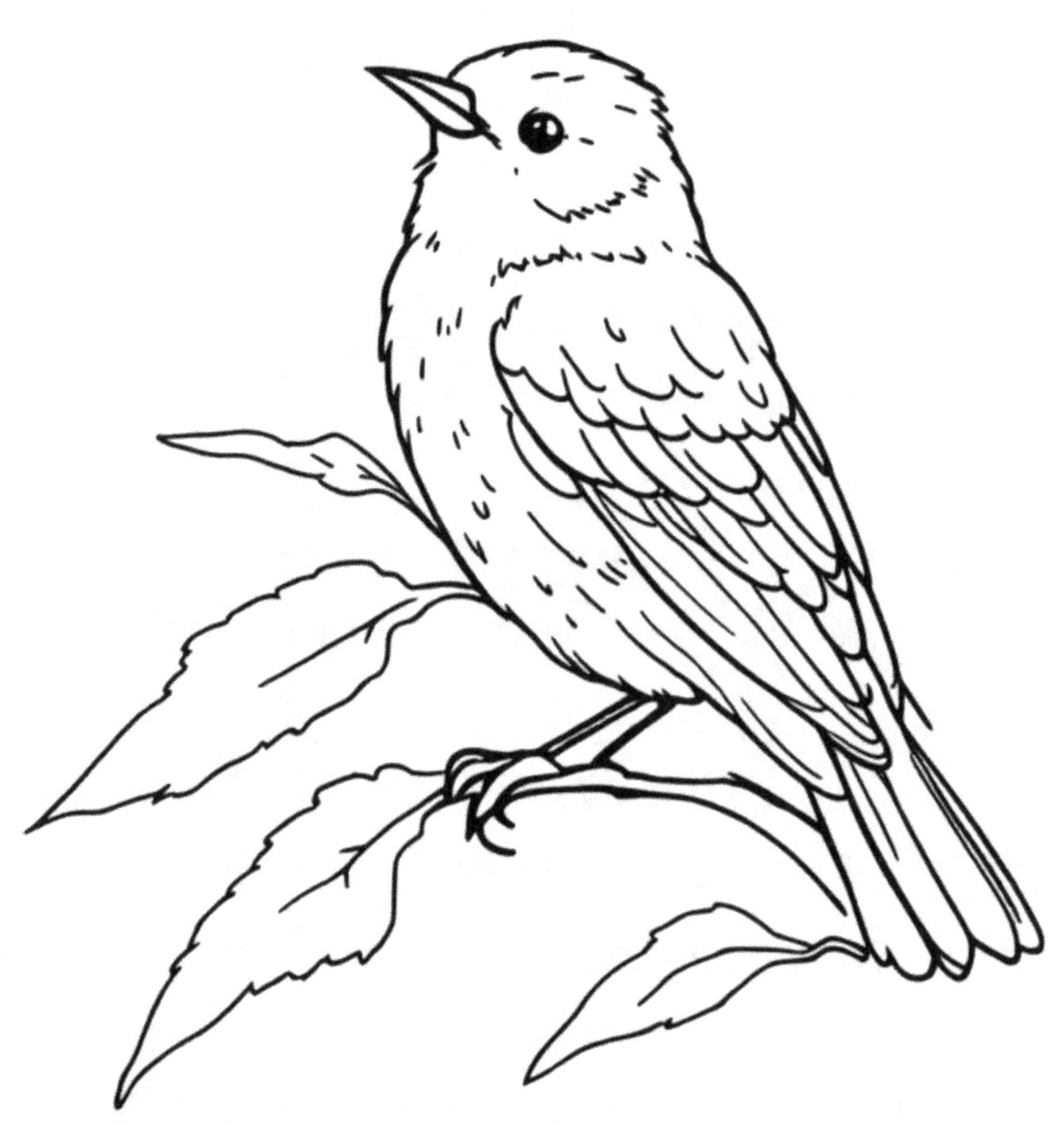

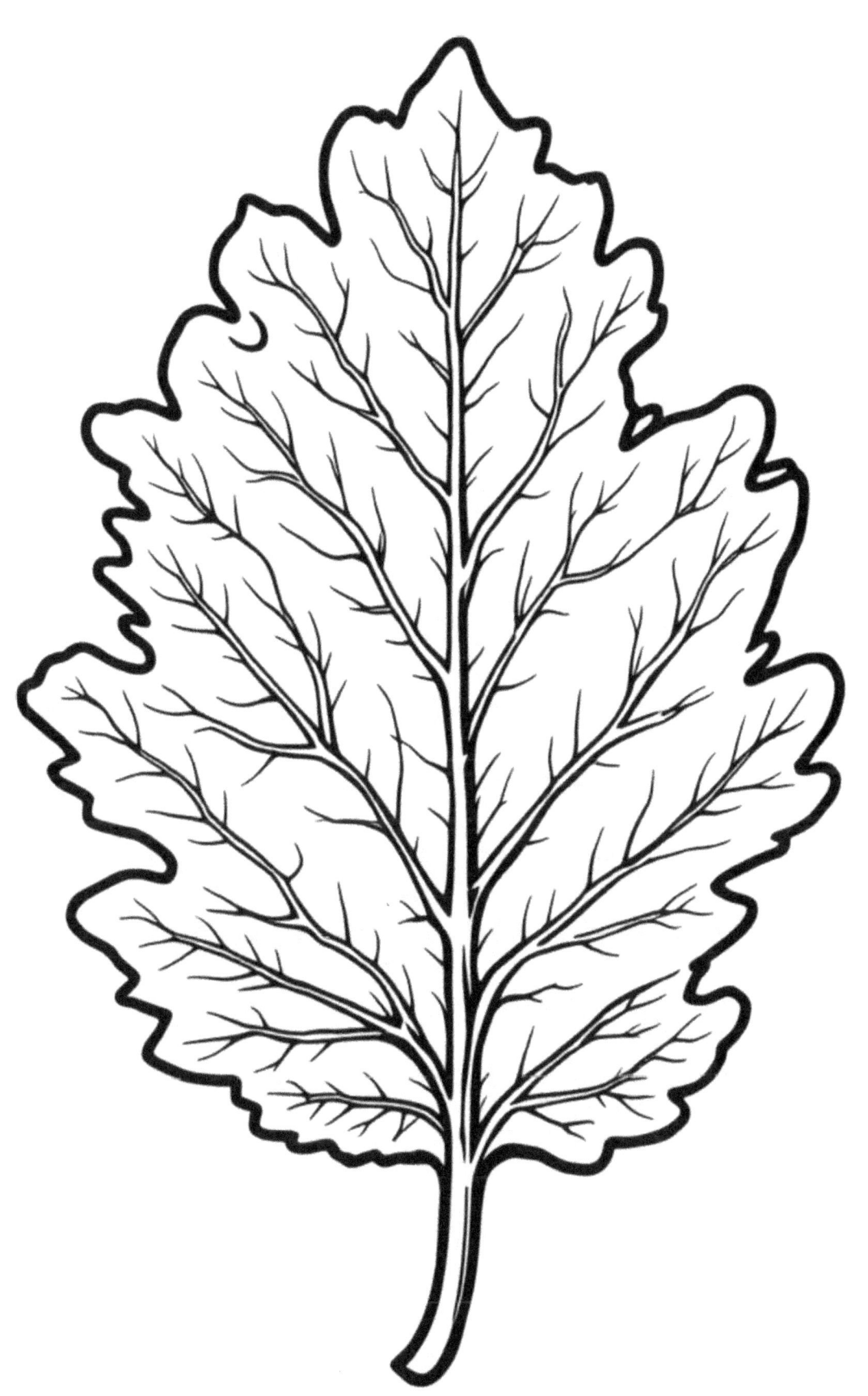

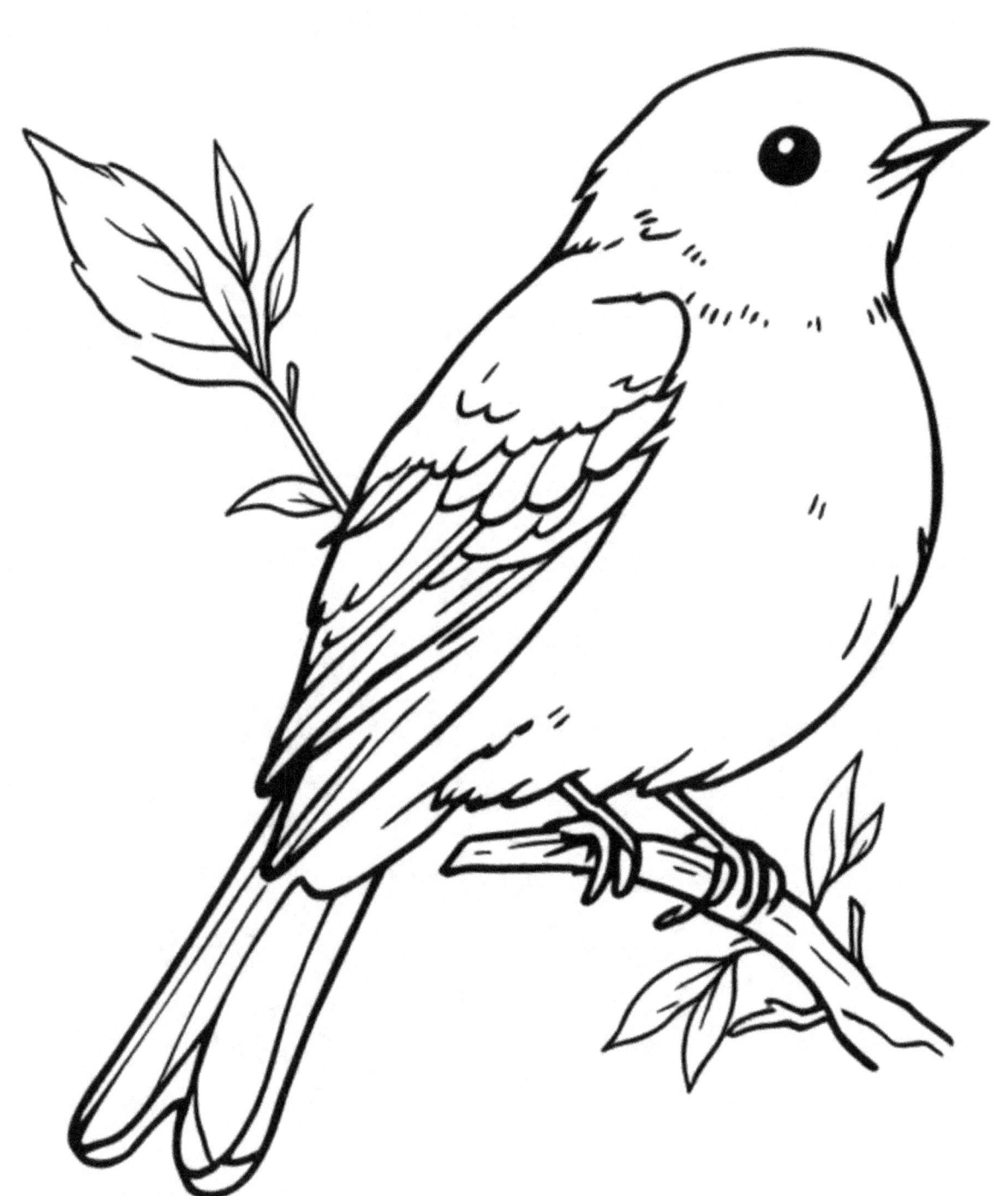

Home & Comfort
(Warm familiarity, reminiscence triggers)

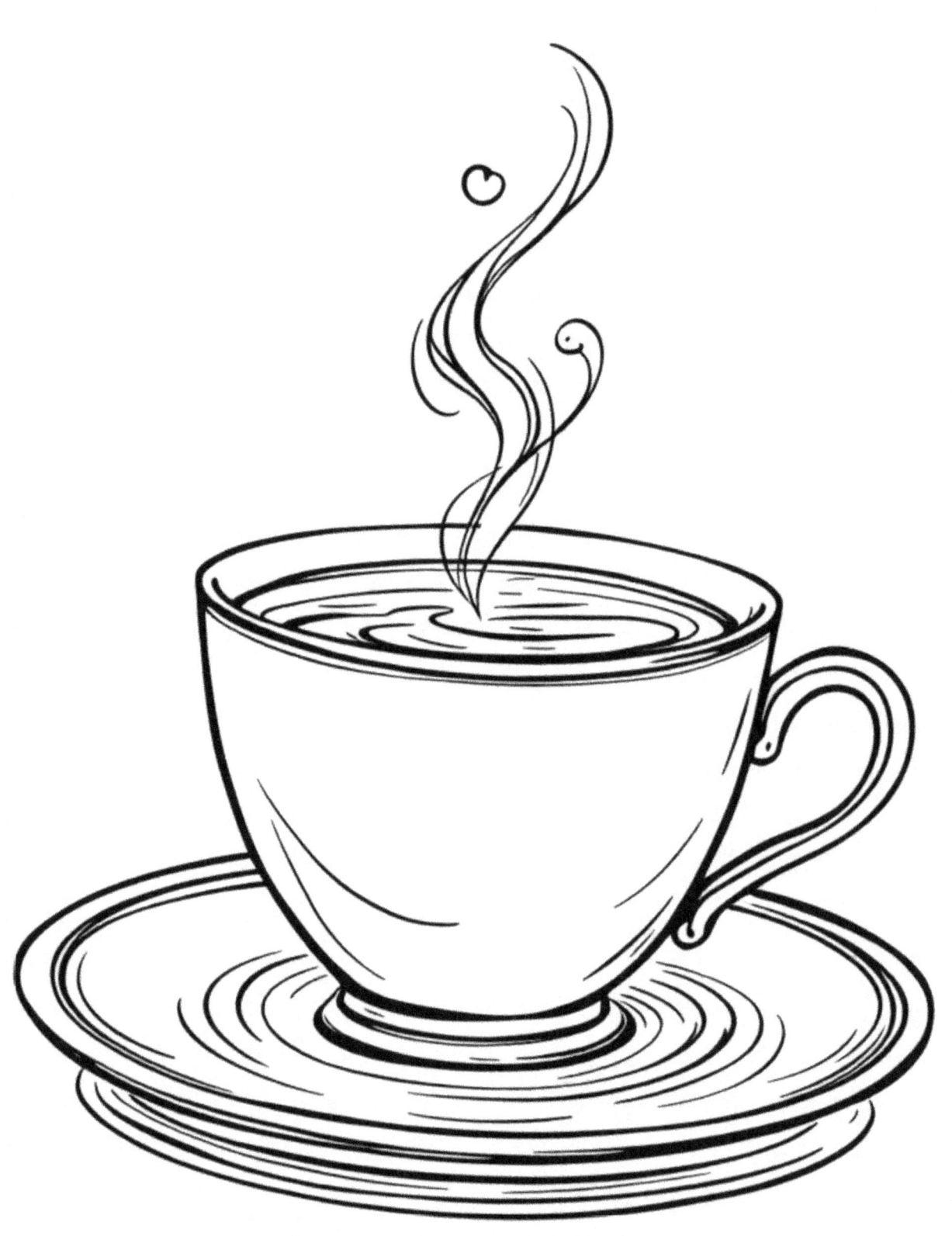

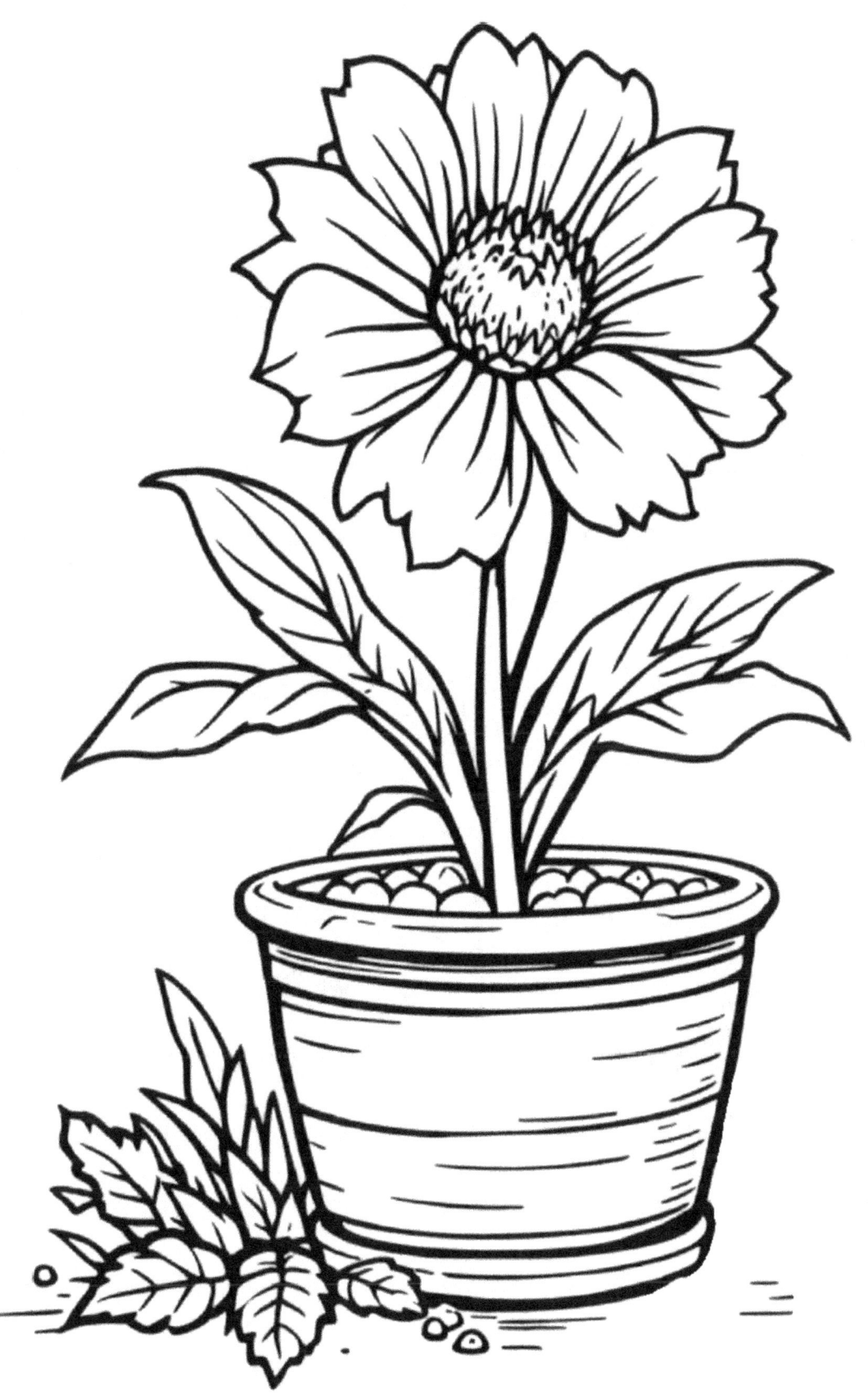

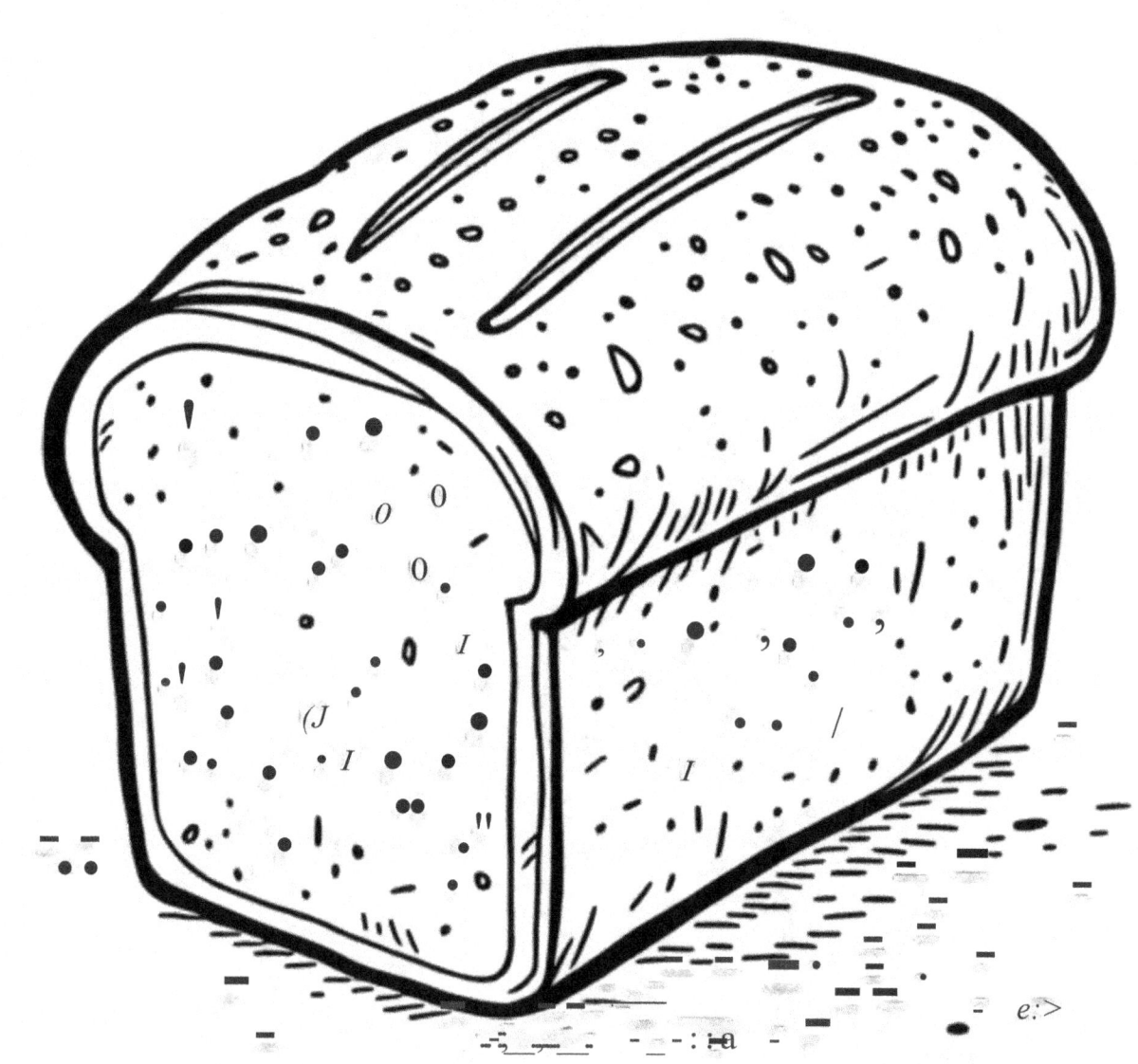

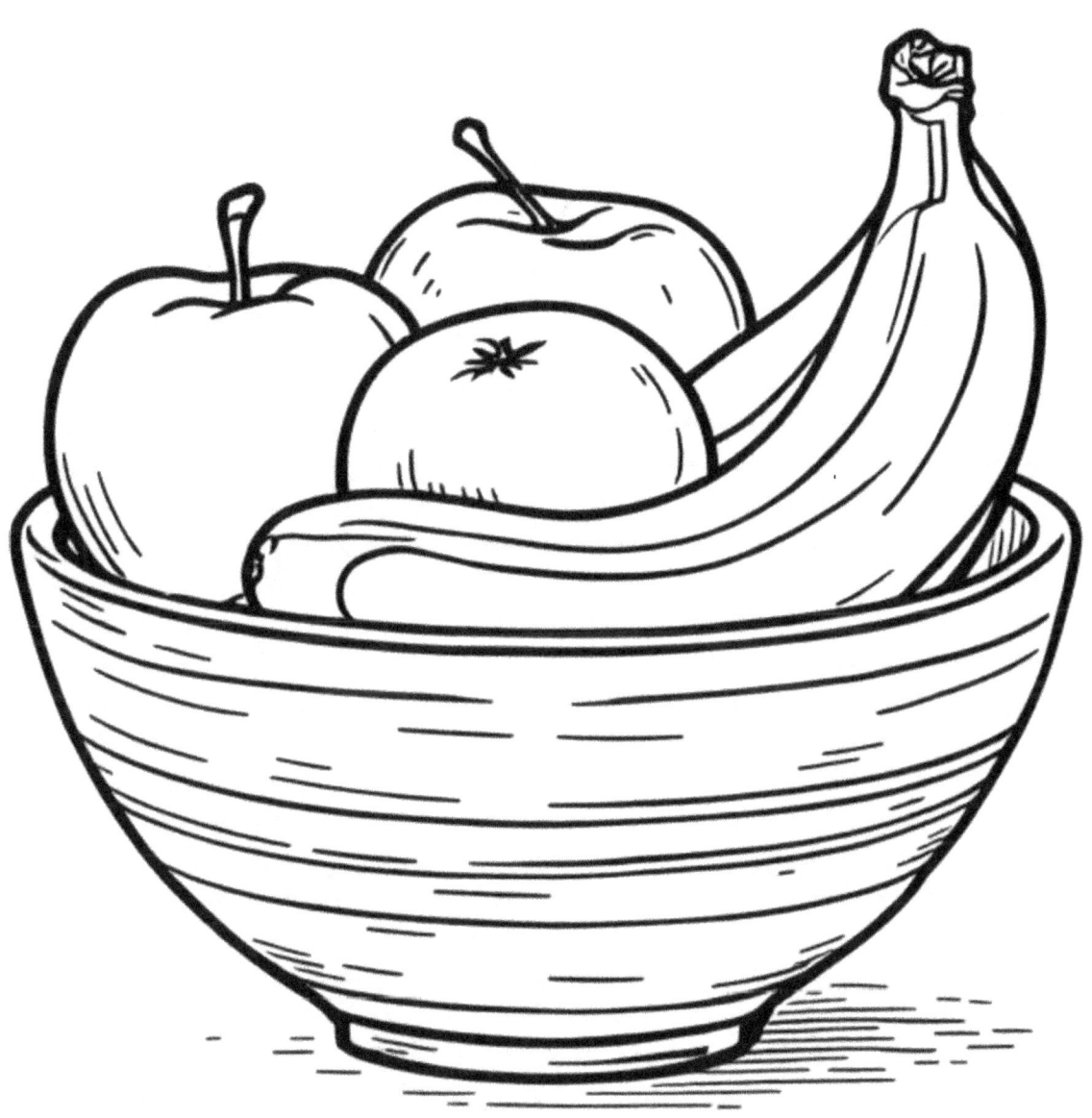

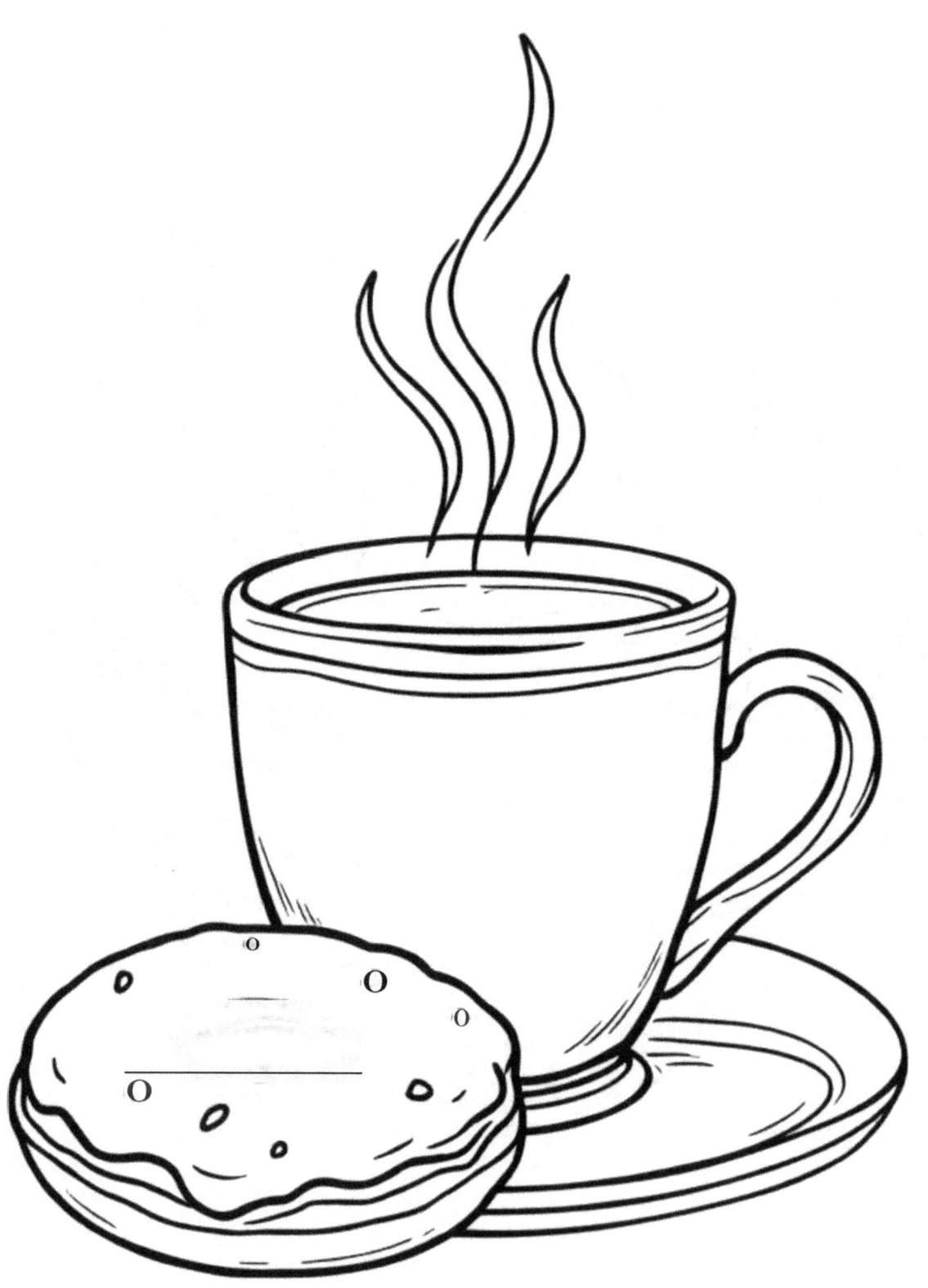

Hobbies & Everyday Joy
(Confidence, identity, purpose)

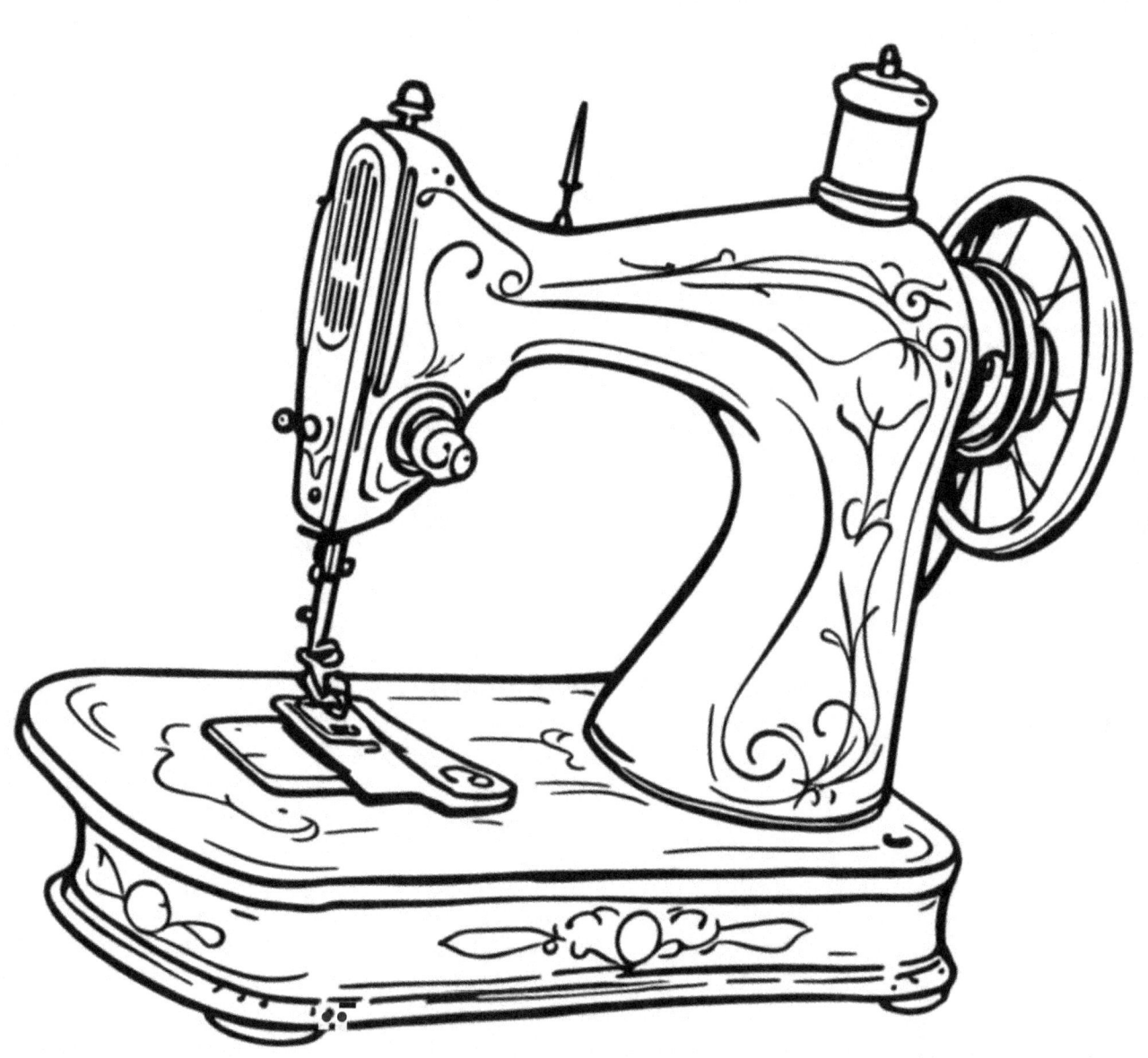

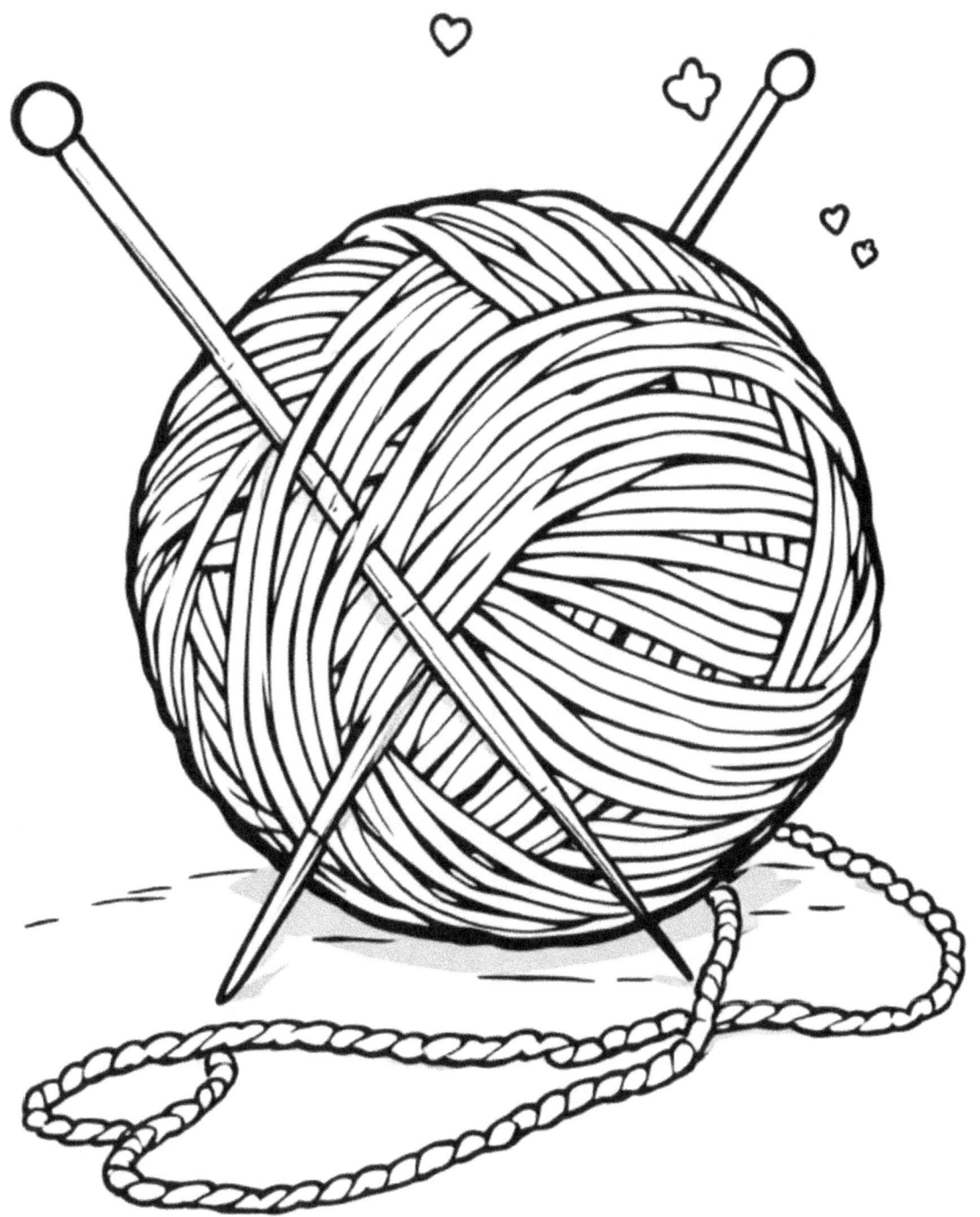

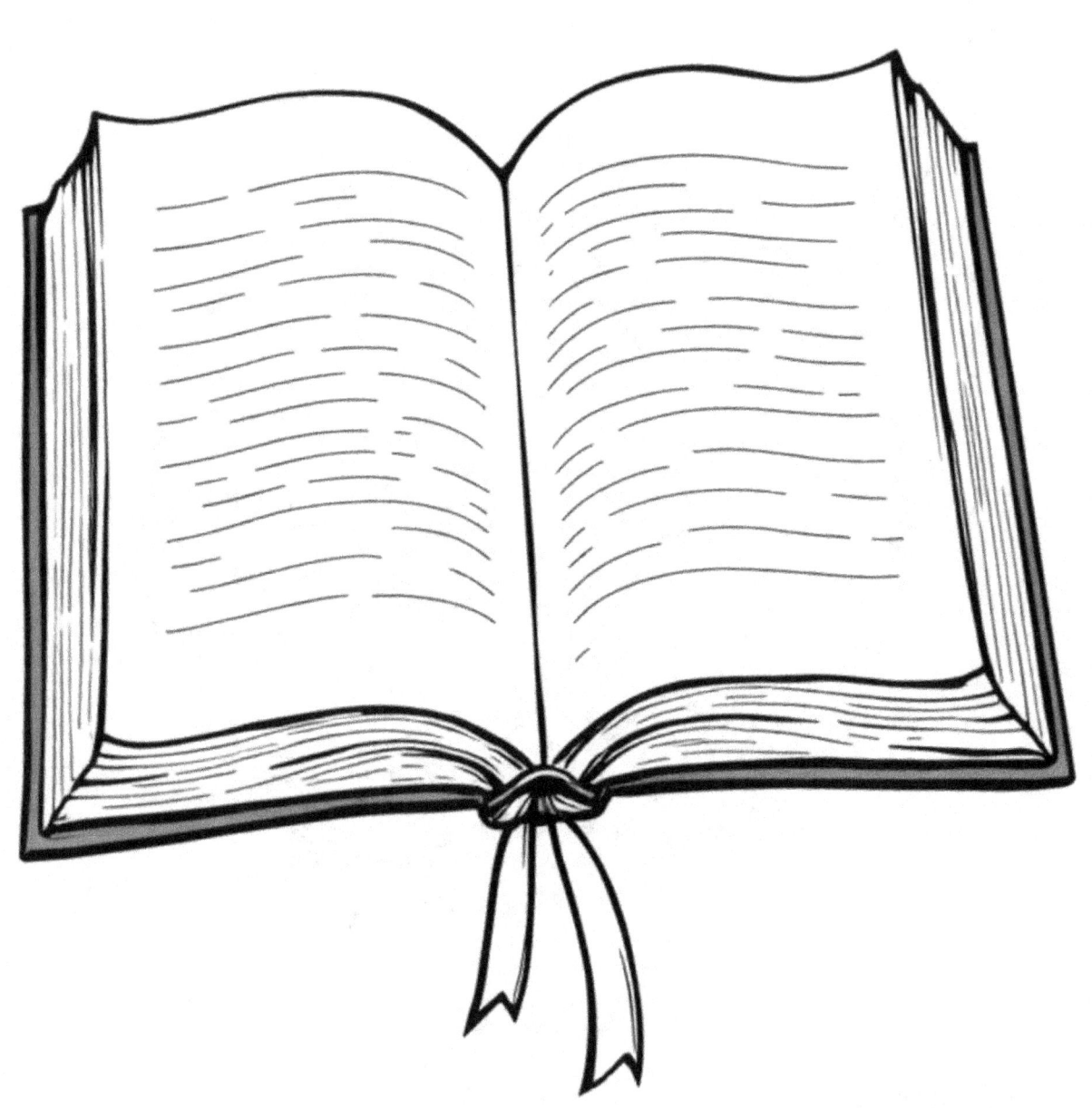

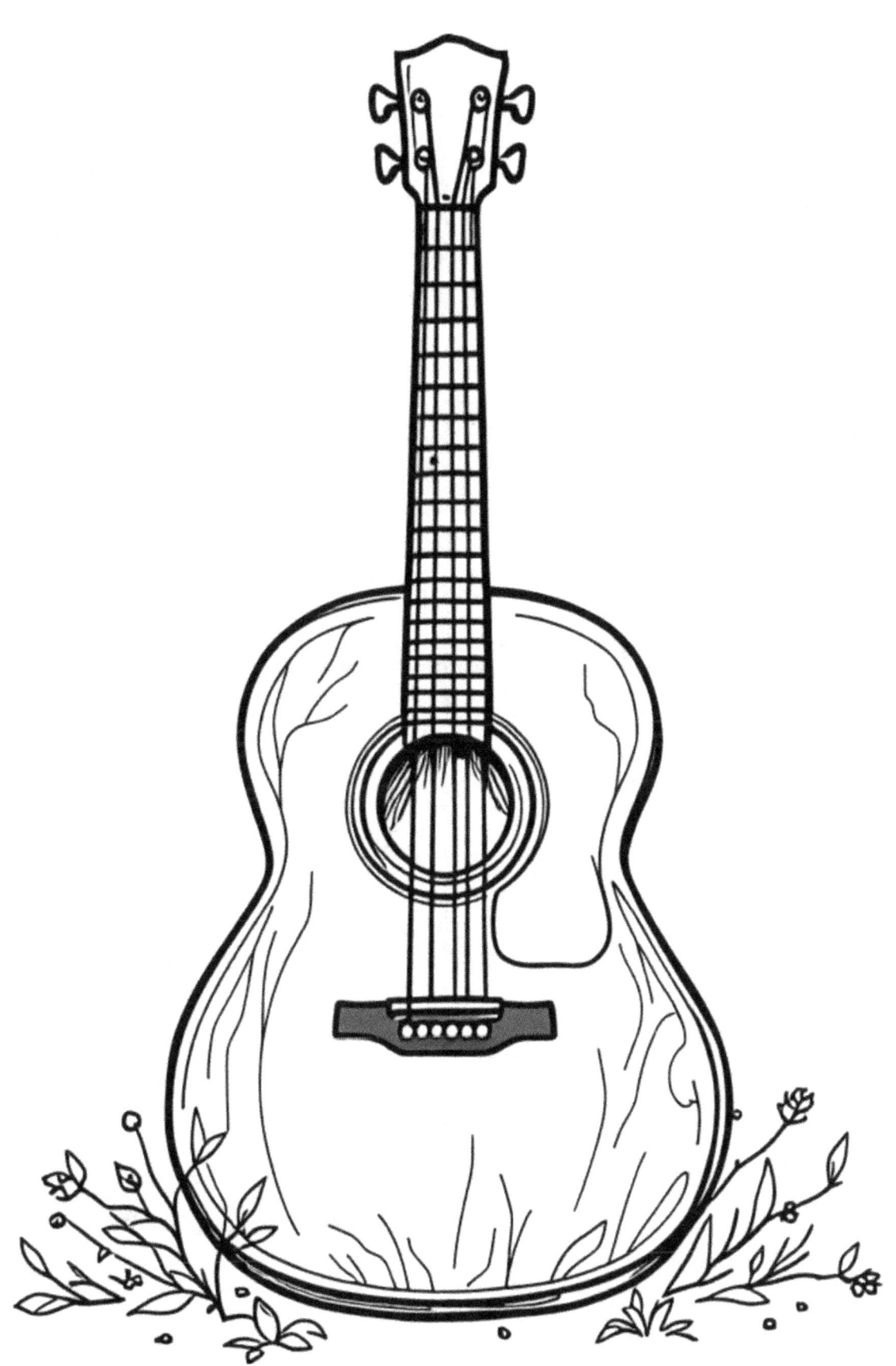

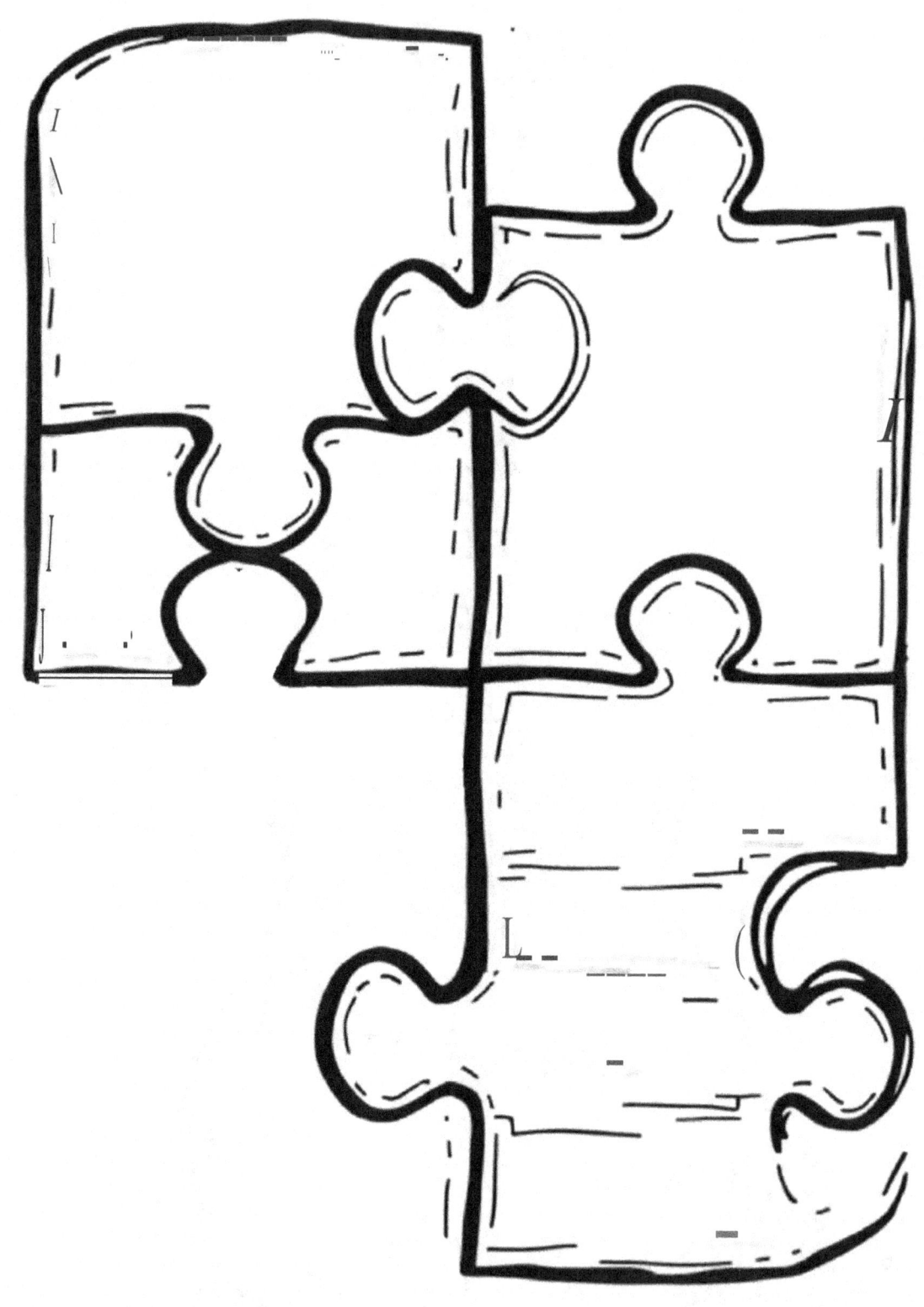

Nostalgia & Memories
(Reminiscence prompts, positive recall)

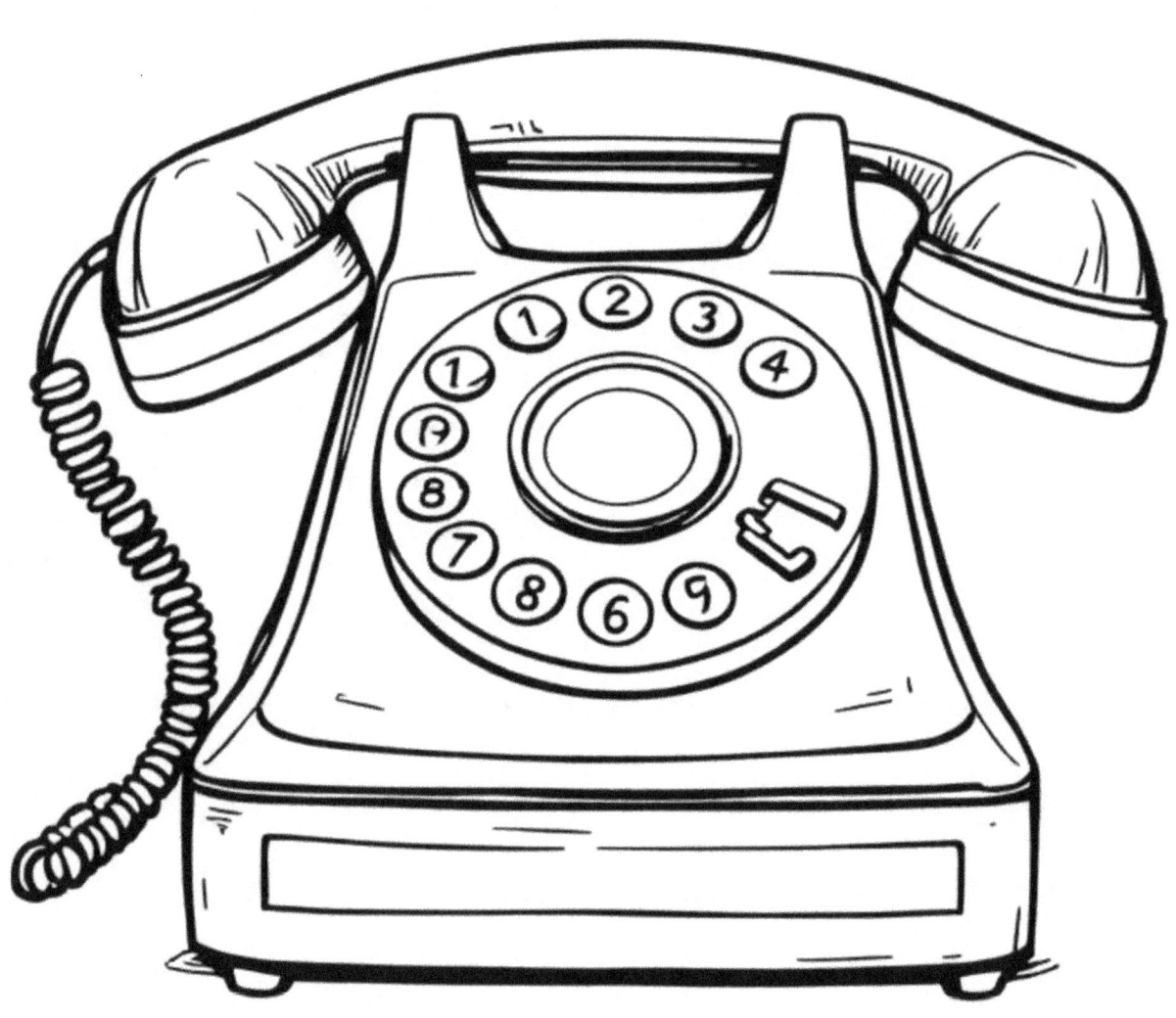

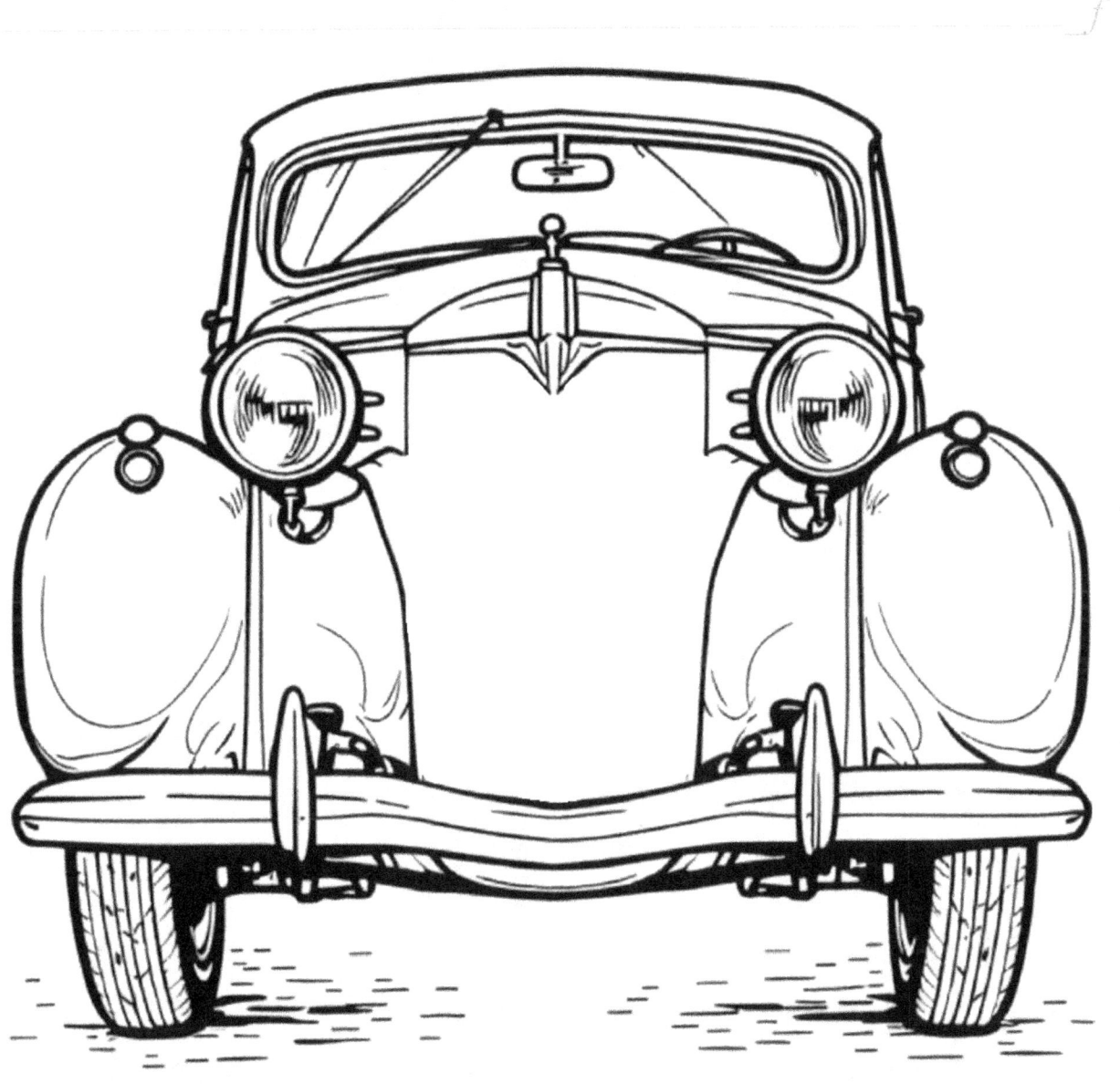

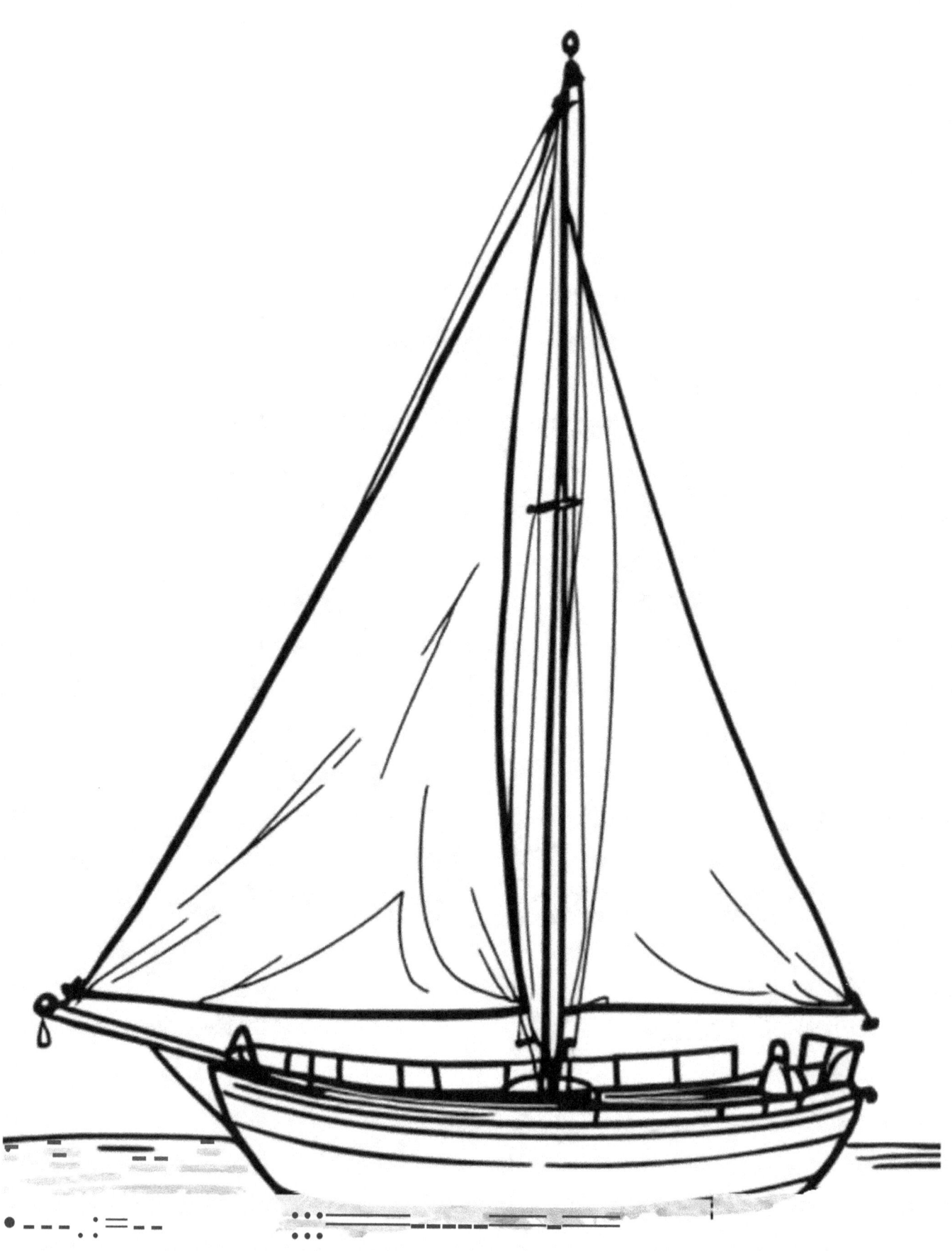

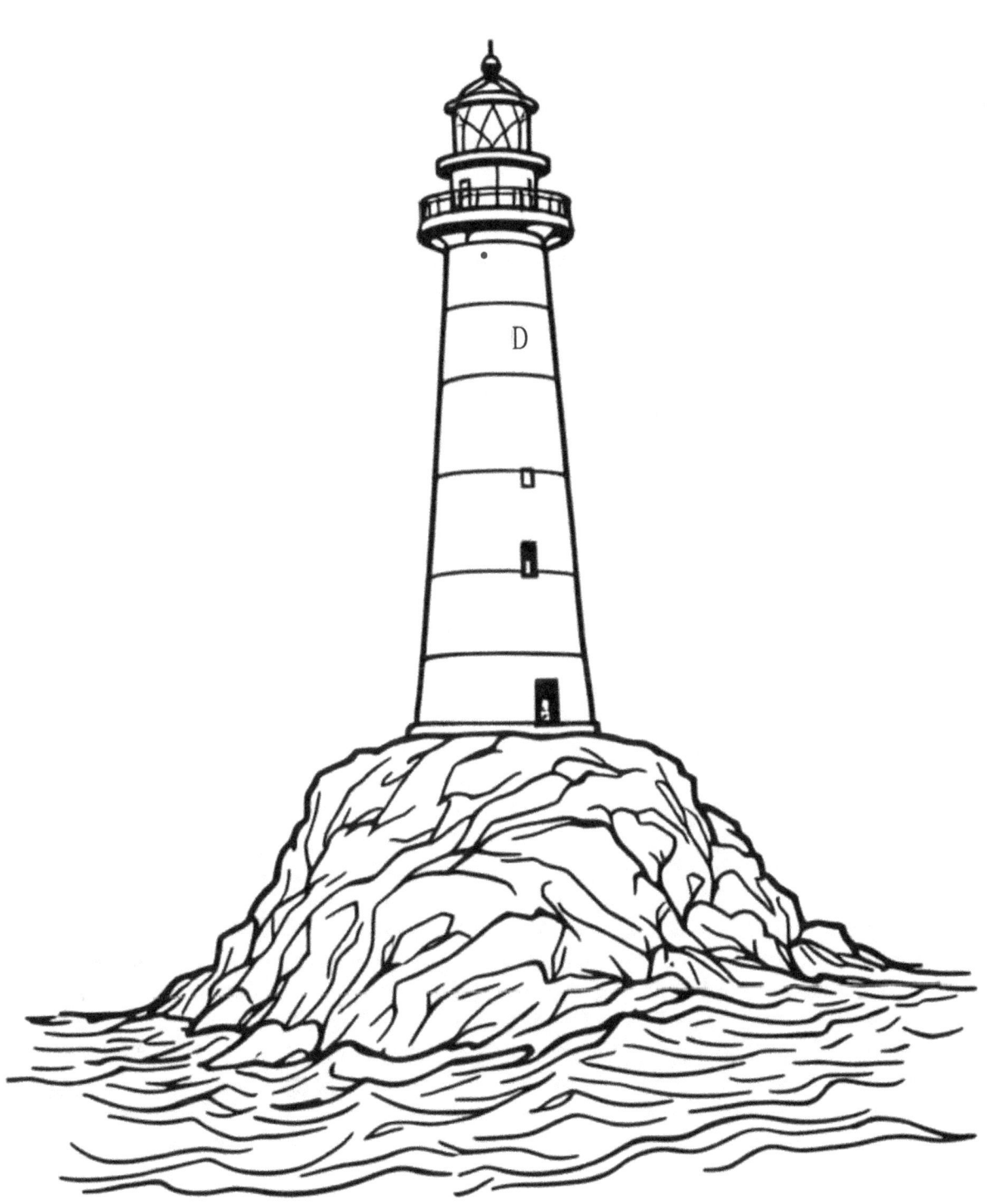

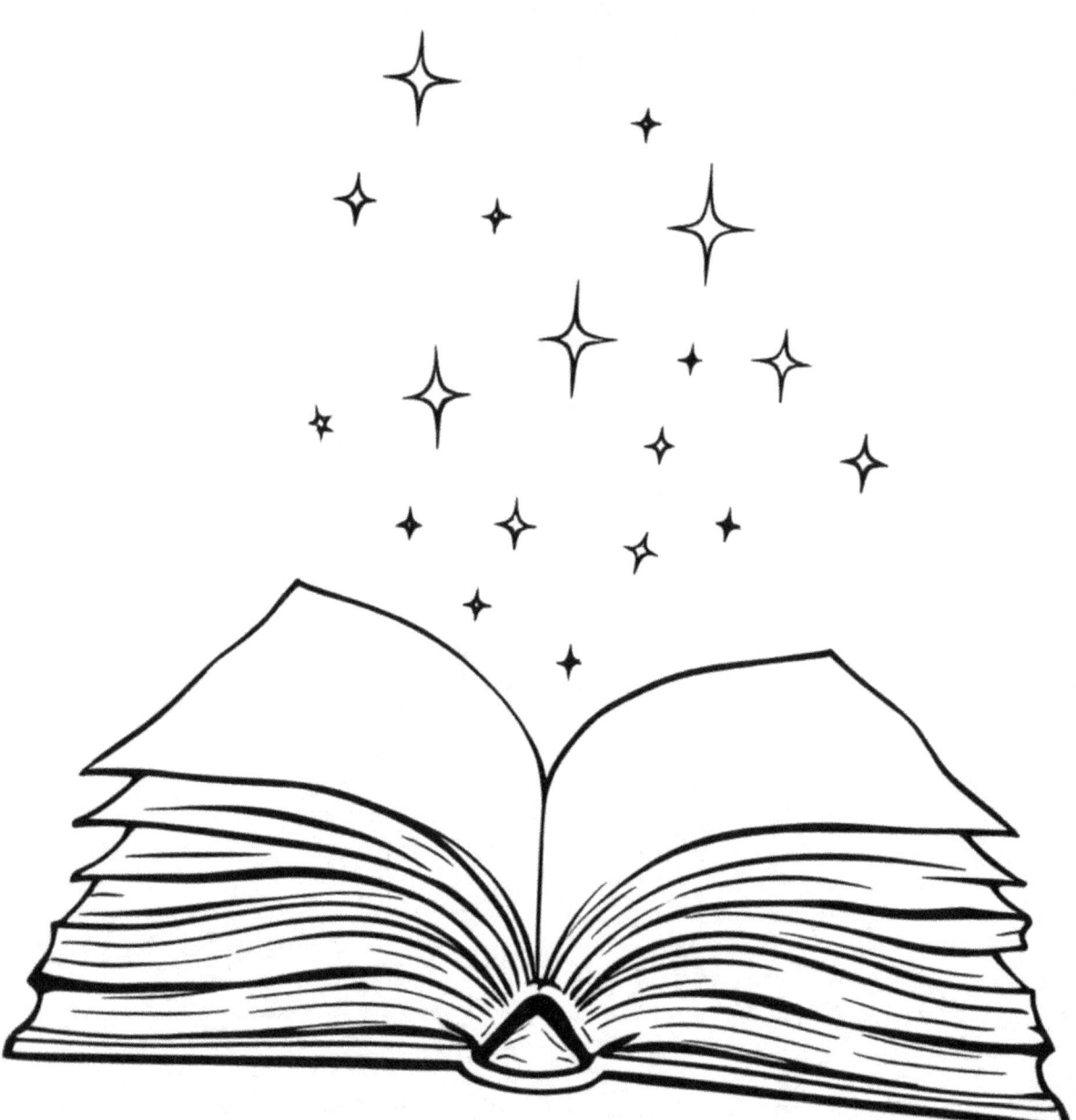

Seasons & Celebration
(Simple joy, rhythm of time)

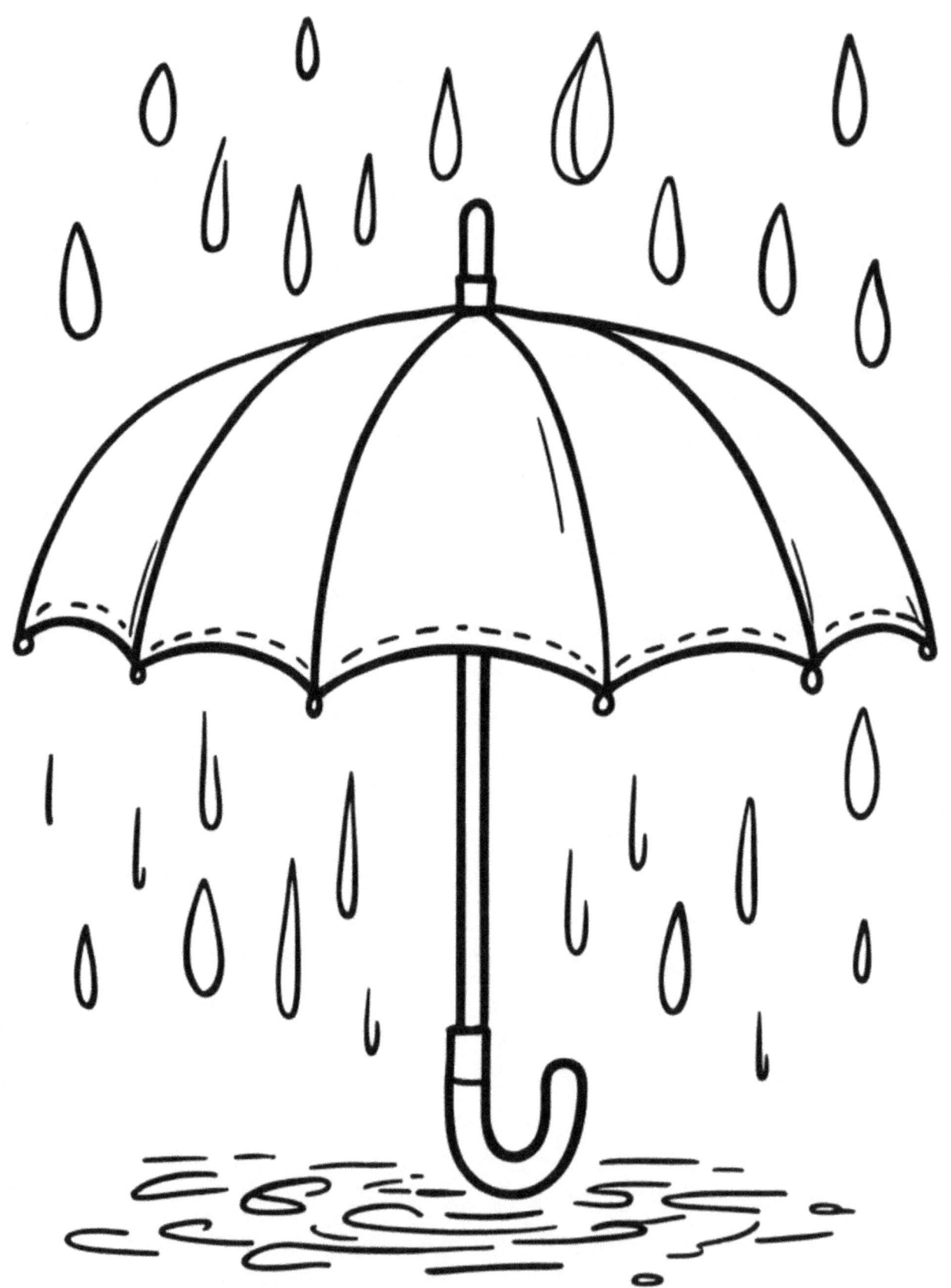

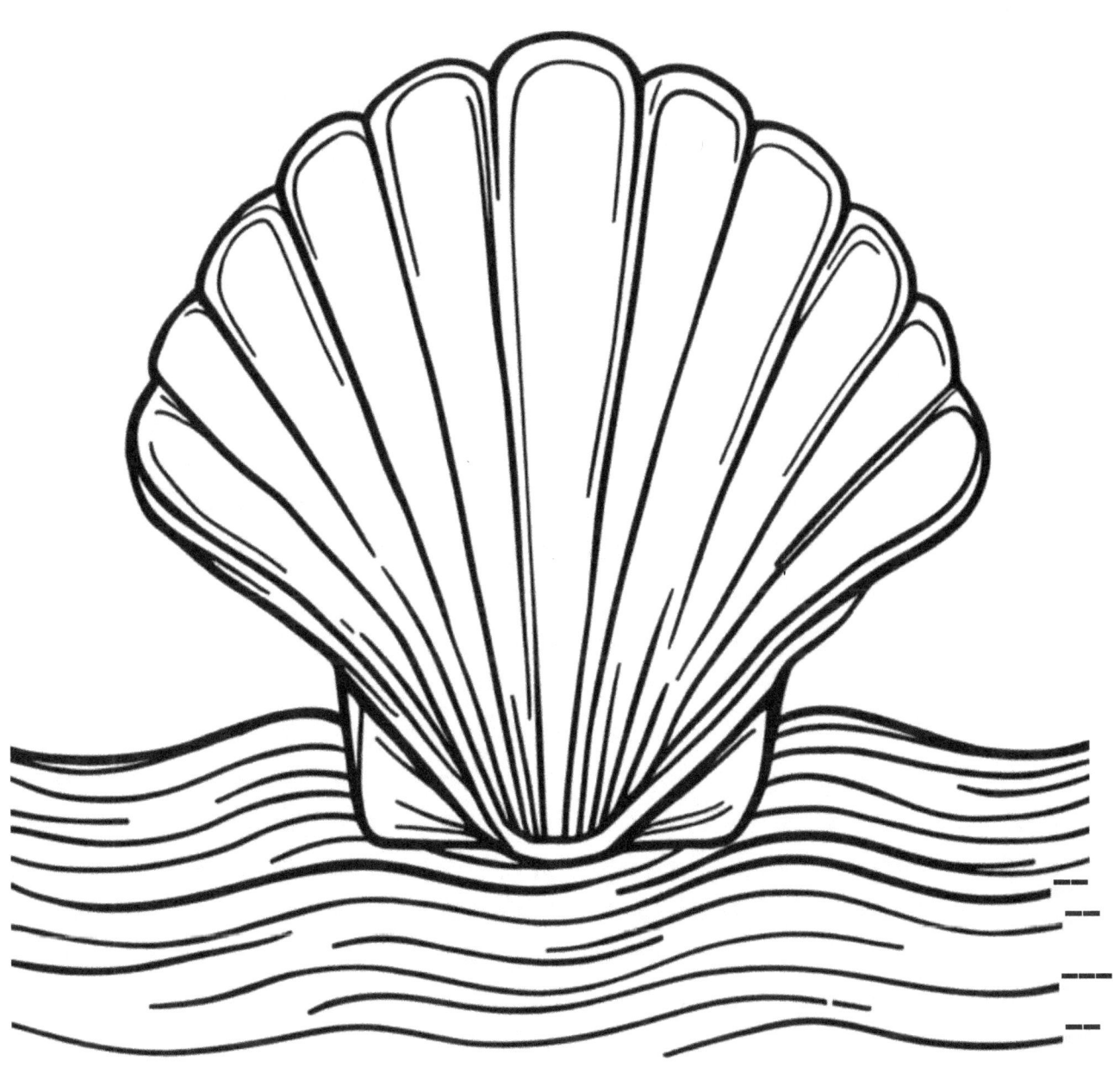

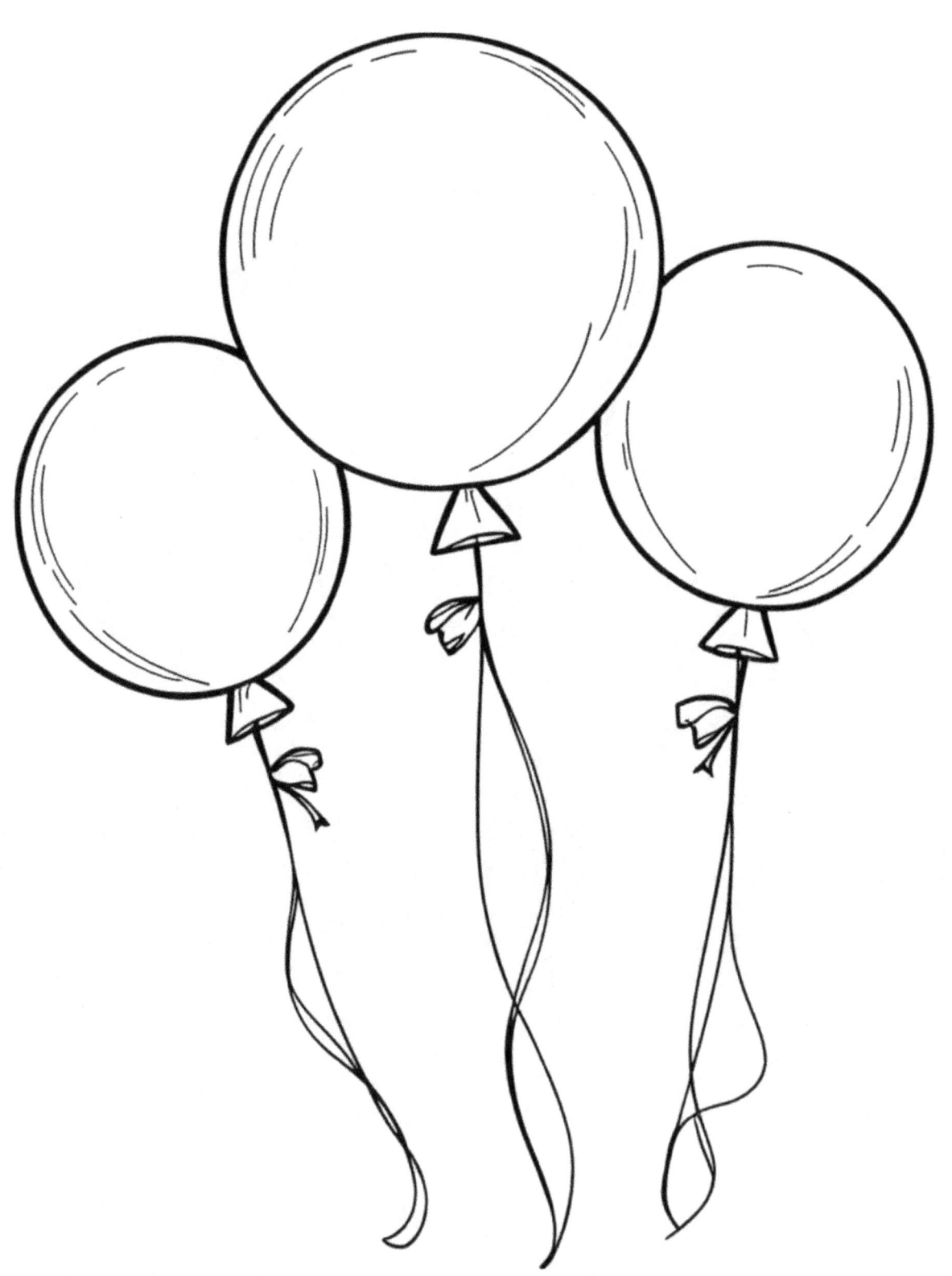

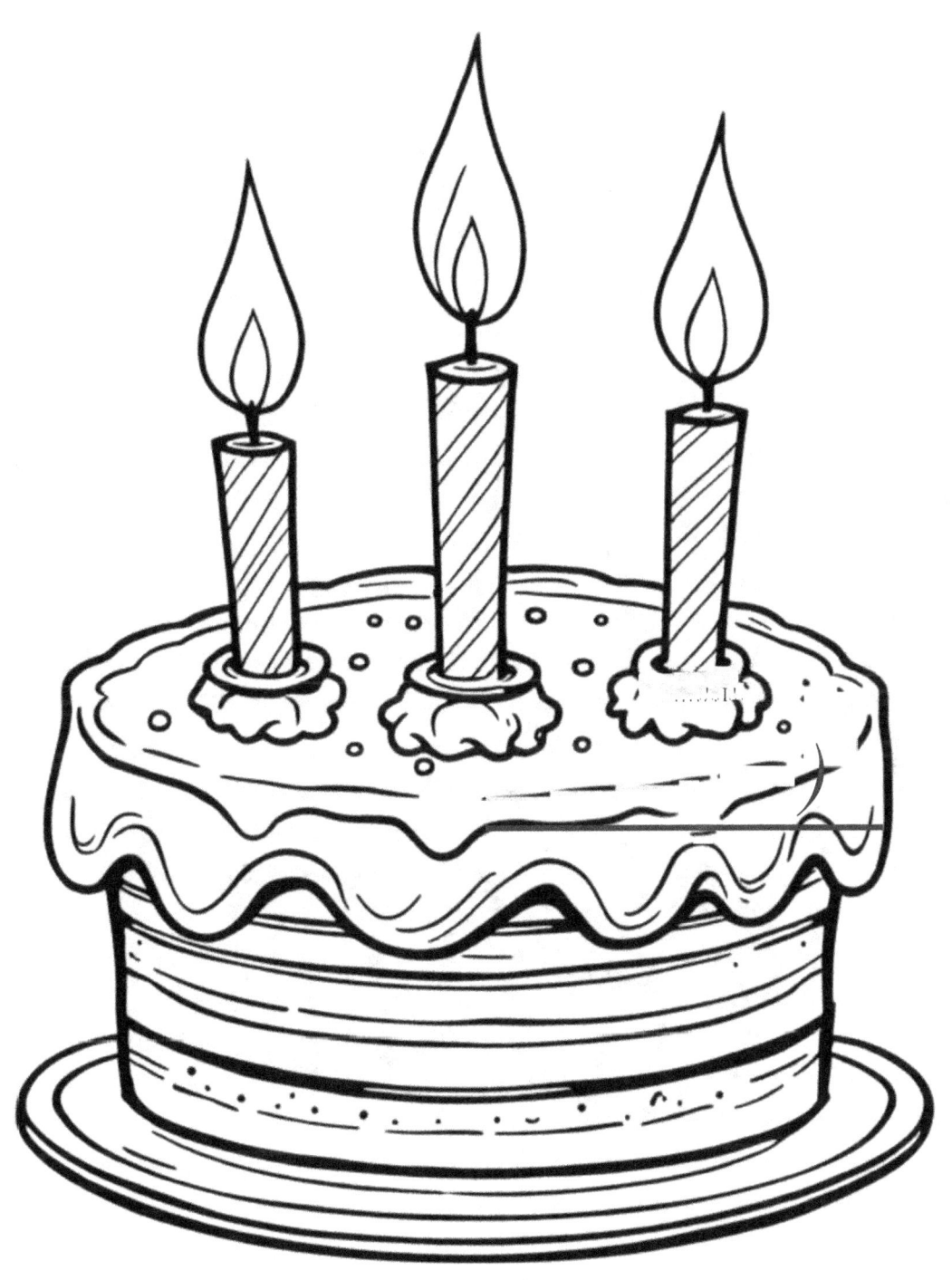

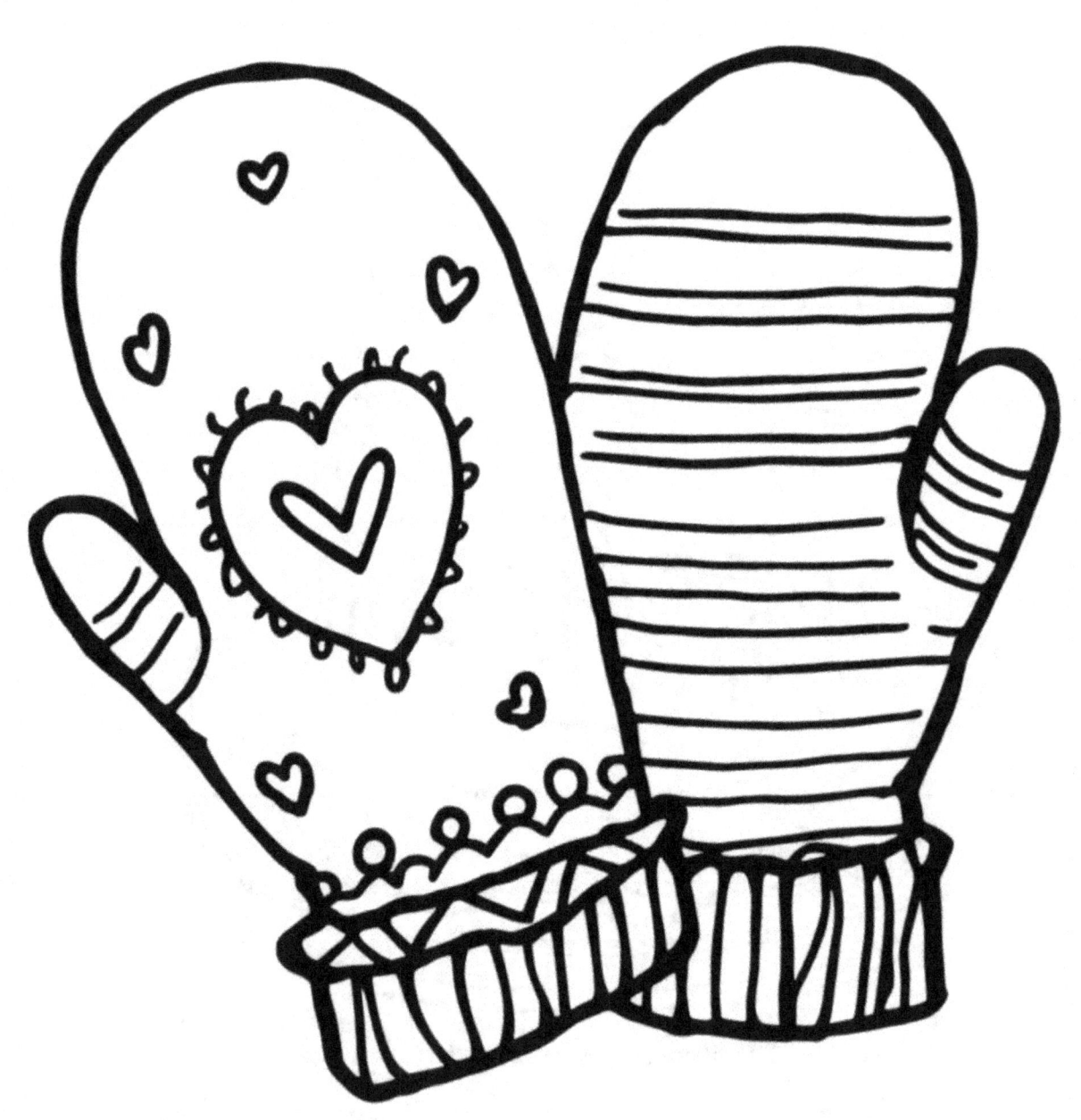

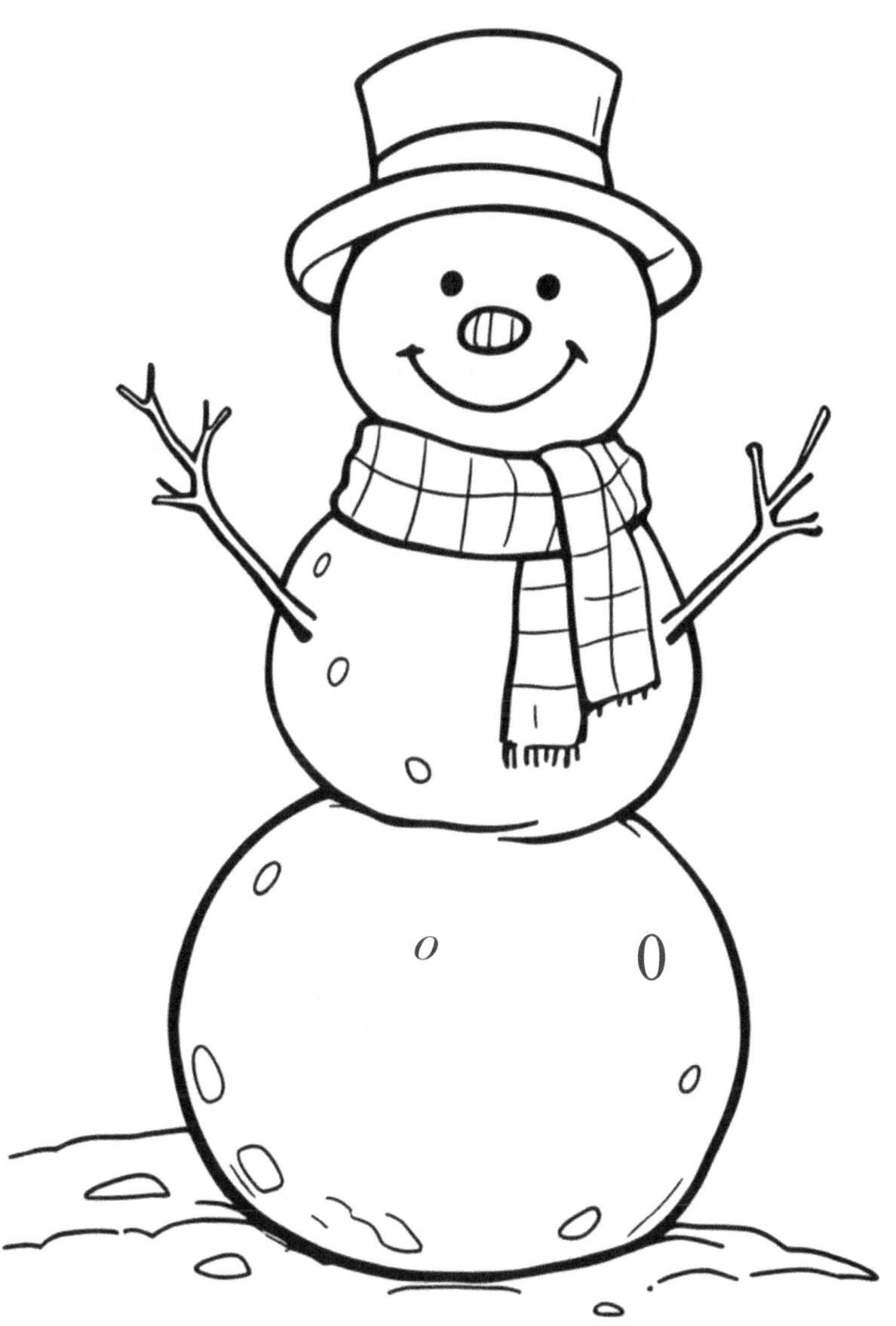

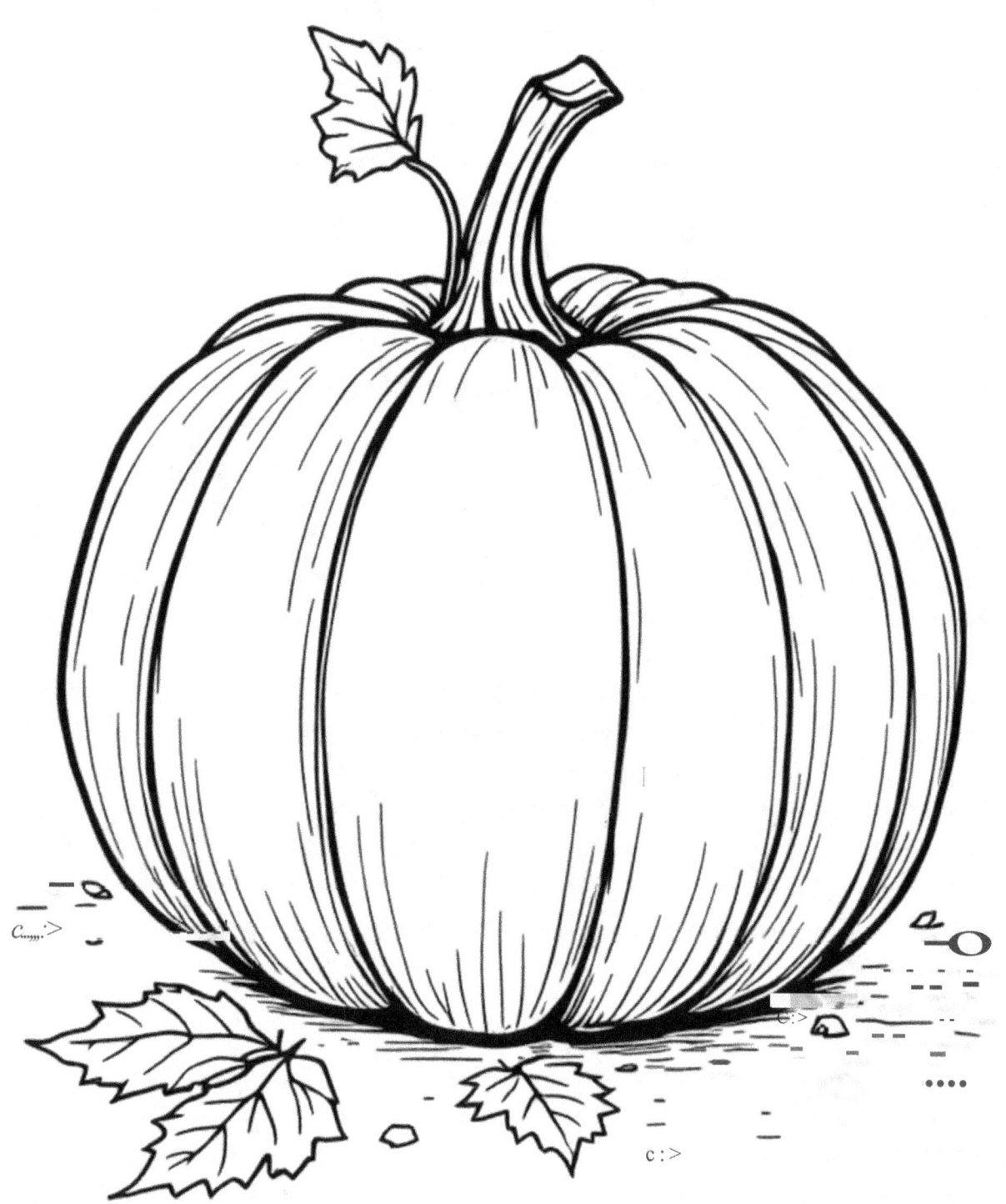

Positivity & Relaxation
(Closing, uplifting finish)

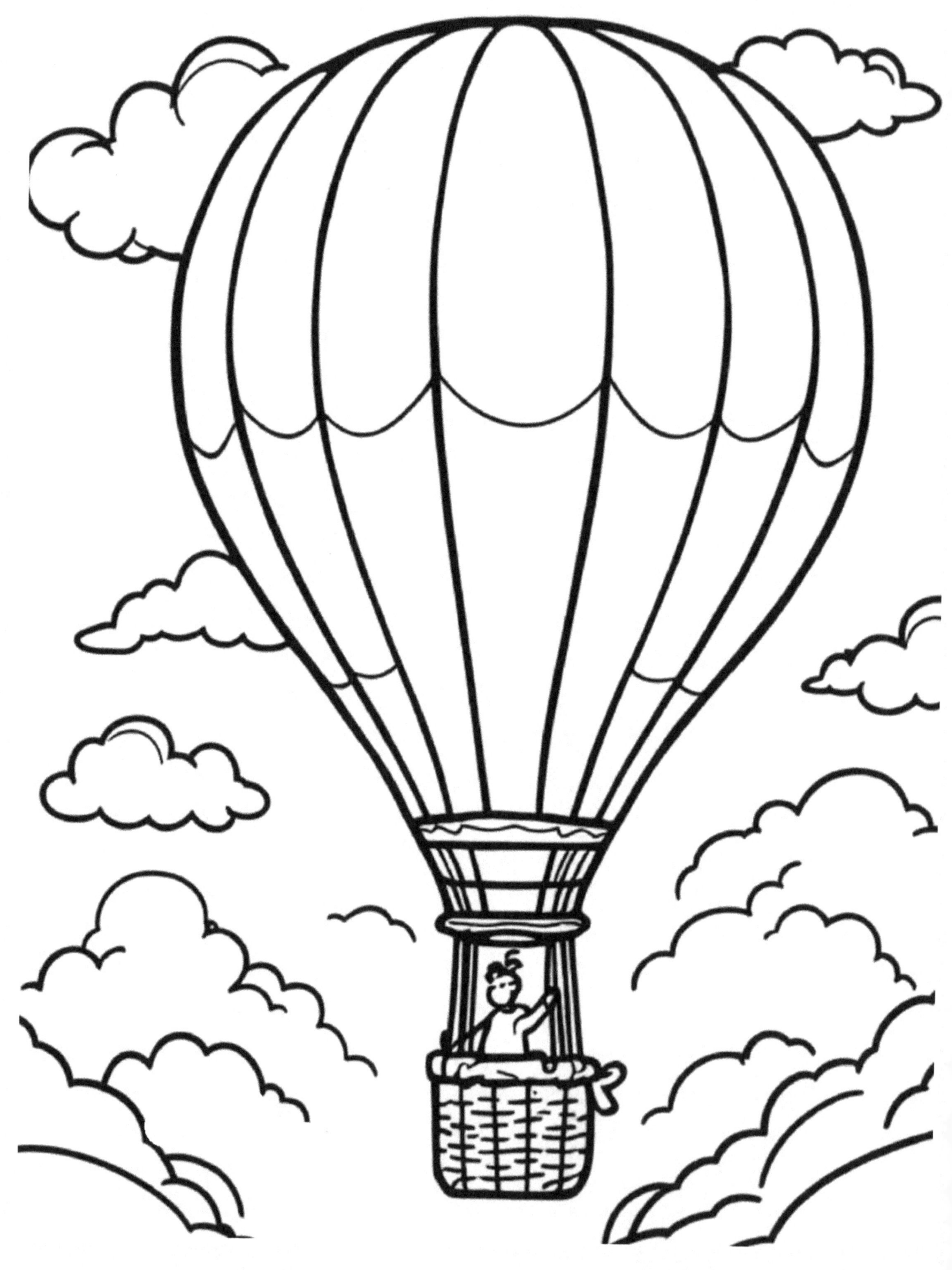

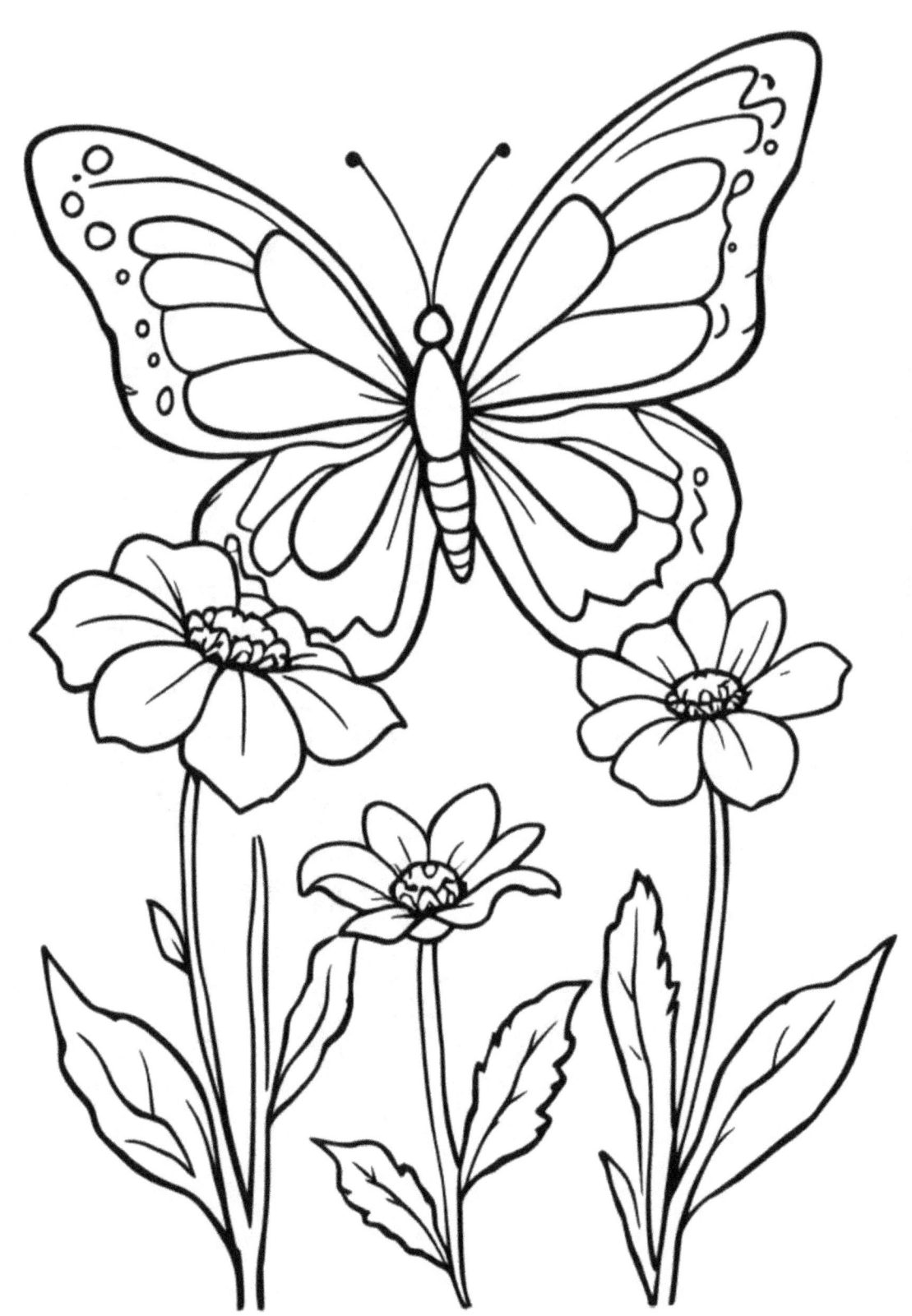

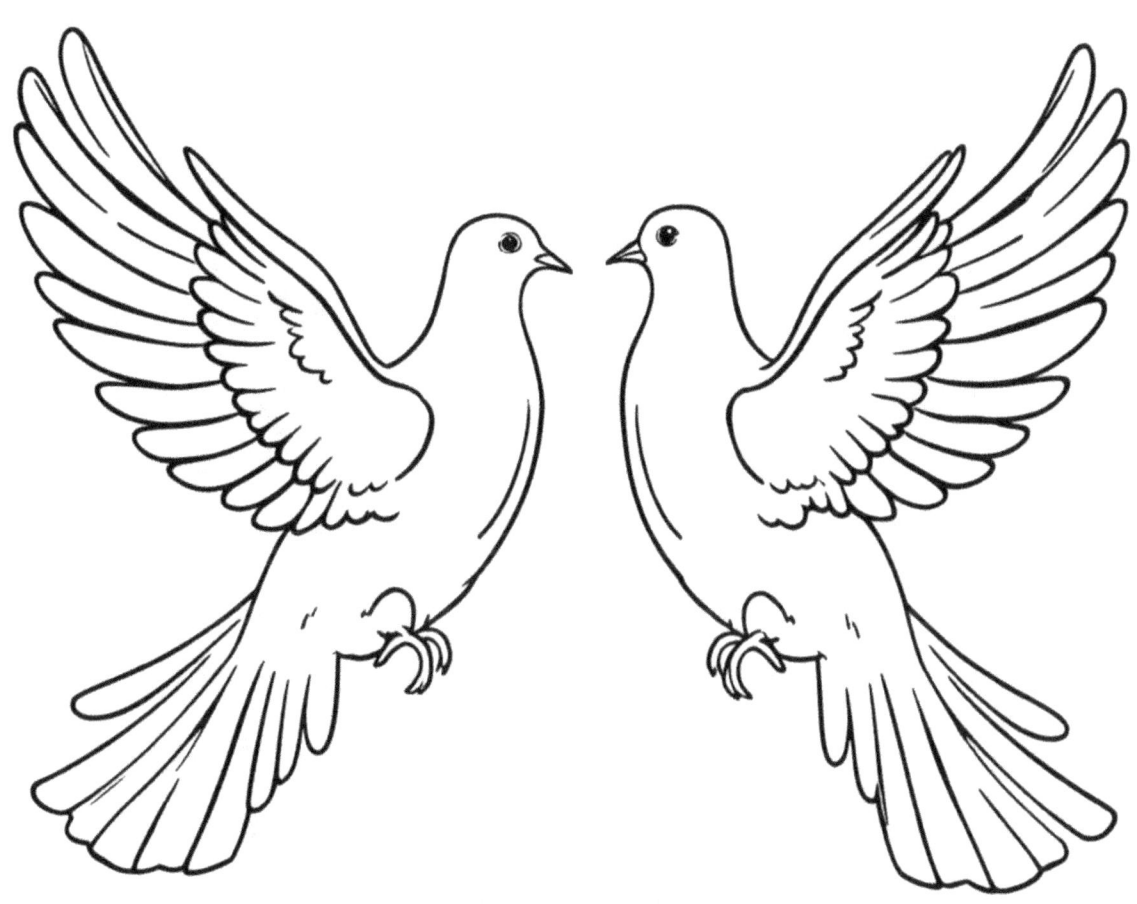

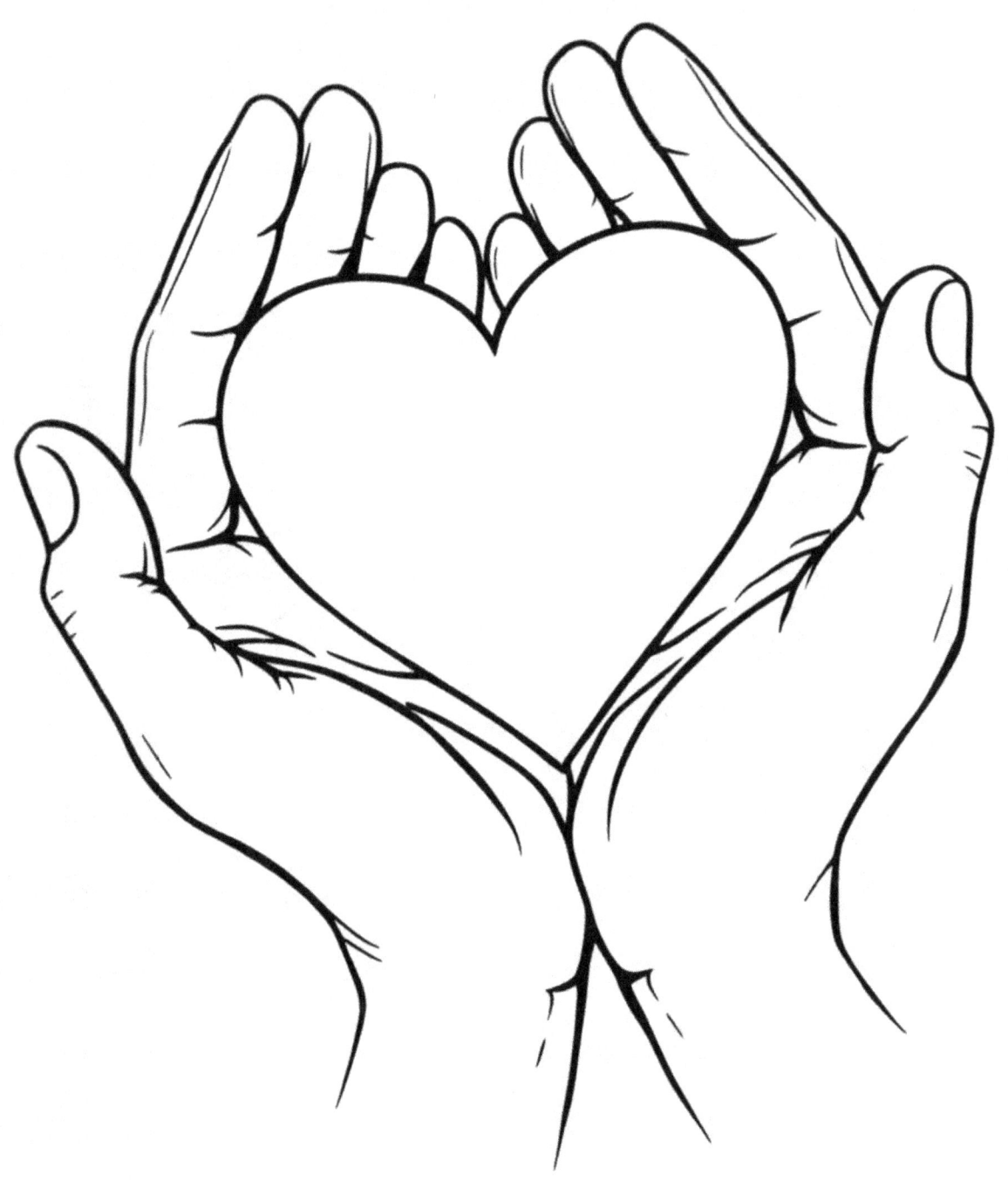

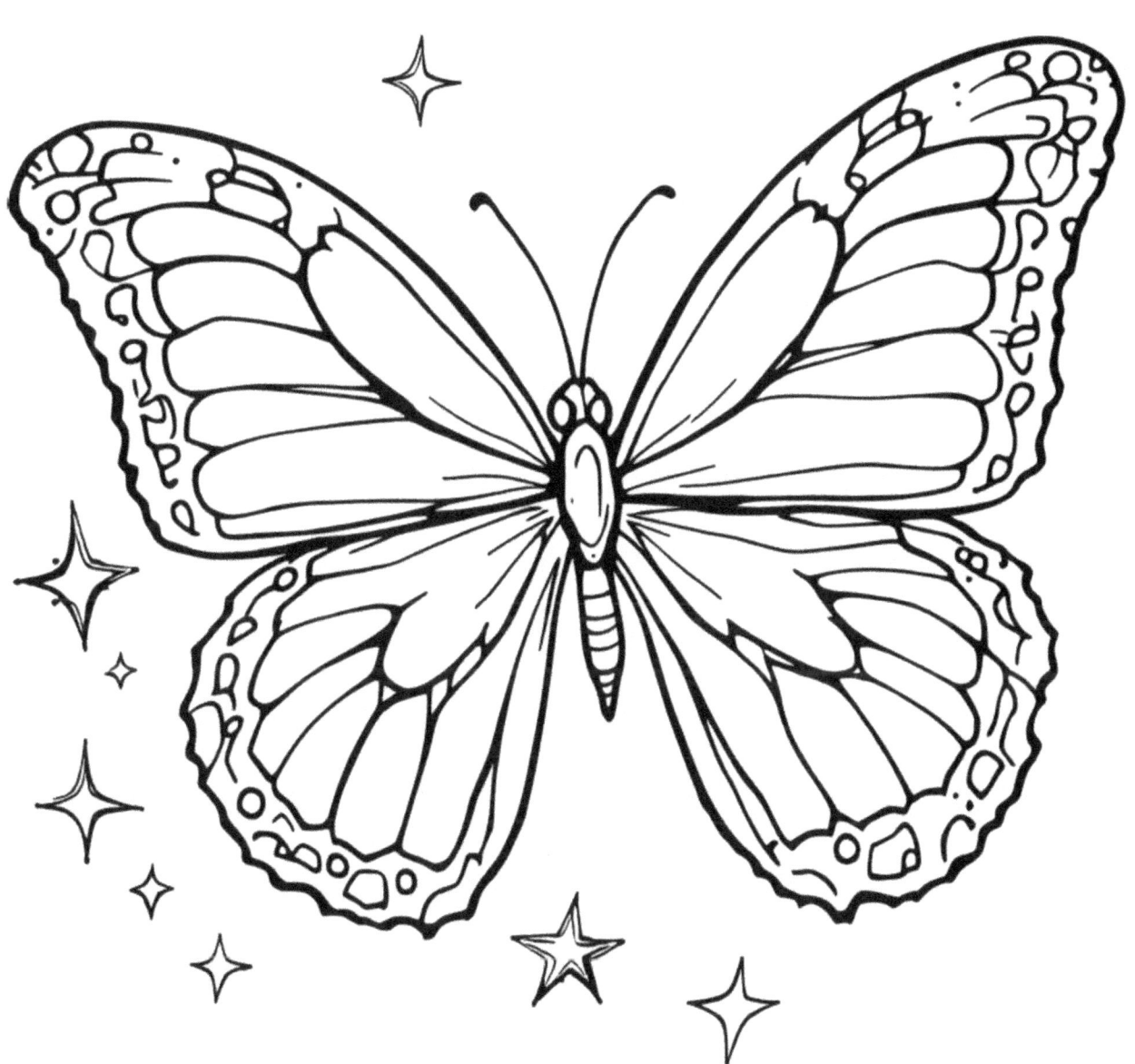

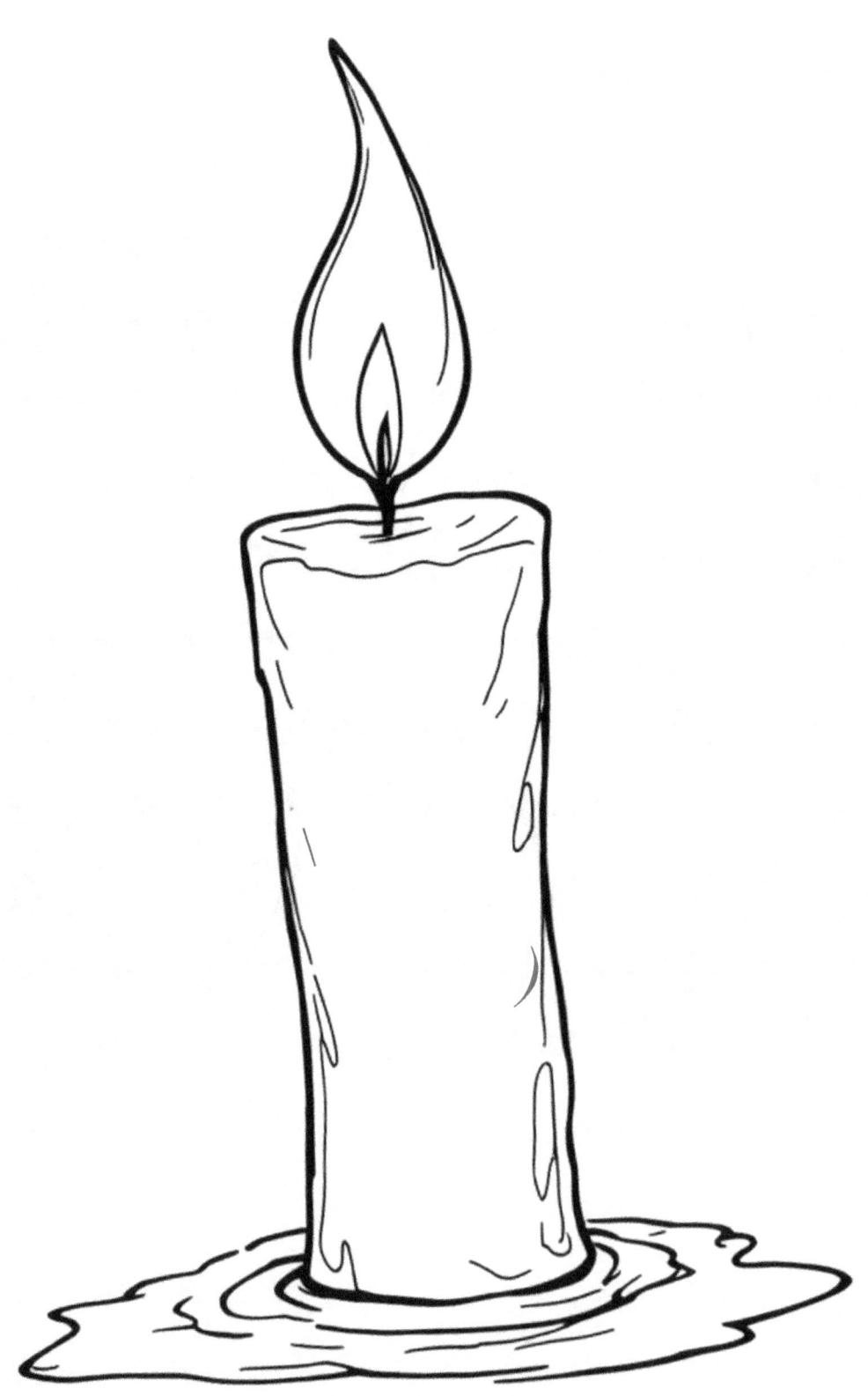

1. Welcome to Your Coloring Book of Calm and Joy

Coloring is a gentle, creative activity that brings calm, focus, and comfort.

For many people, especially older adults and those living with memory loss, coloring feels familiar and reassuring. The simple act of choosing a color and filling a shape can help quiet the mind and bring a sense of peace.

This book has been created with care for individuals who benefit from clear, uncomplicated images. Each page offers one large subject with bold outlines and plenty of open white space. There are no tiny patterns or confusing backgrounds - just simple, happy designs that invite success and enjoyment.

Family members, caregivers, and activity coordinators can use this book as a shared moment of connection. There is no right or wrong way to color. The goal is not perfection—it is enjoyment, relaxation, and comfort.

Whether used at home, in a care facility, or as part of an activity group, this book is meant to bring small moments of happiness and calm to everyone who opens it.

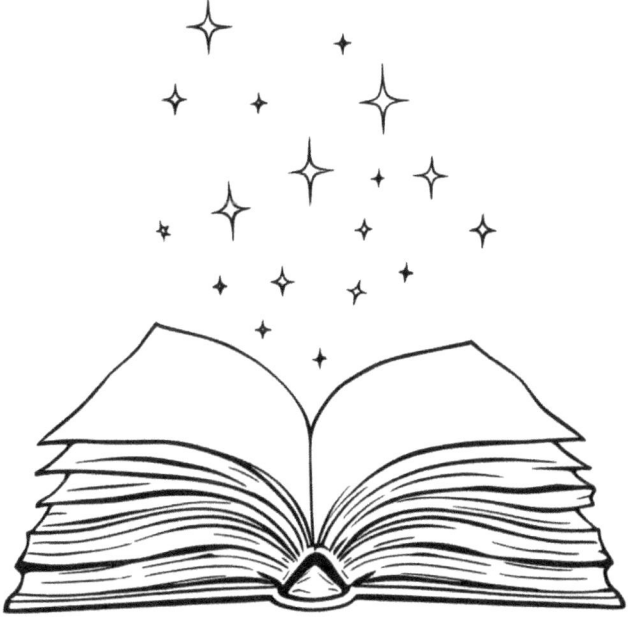

2. How to Support a Loved One While Coloring

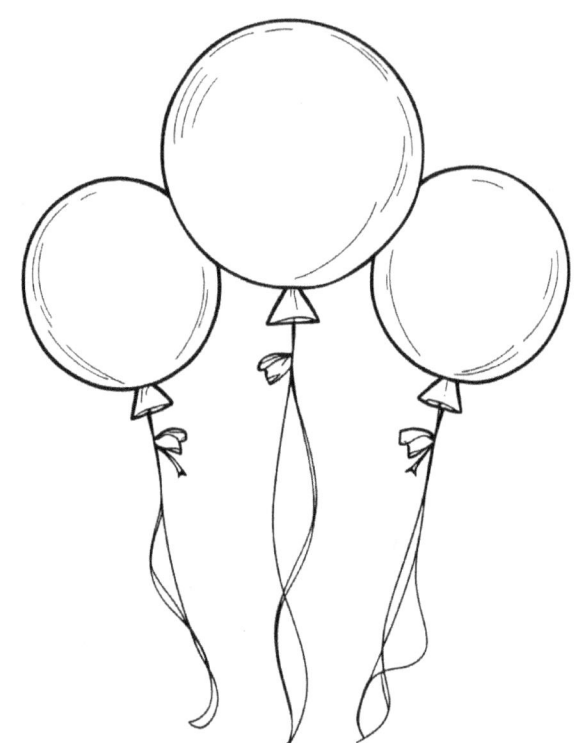

Coloring together can become a special shared time. For many people with dementia or Alzheimer's, familiar routines help them feel secure. Here are some gentle suggestions for making this activity meaningful: Create a calm space. Choose a quiet table with good lighting and minimal distractions. Play soft music if it helps set a relaxing mood.

Offer clear choices. Present two or three colors at a time rather than the entire box of pencils. Too many options can feel confusing.

Encourage, don't correct. There is no "right" color for a cat, a flower, or a house. Let them enjoy choosing colors freely.

Join in if invited. Some people like to color alongside someone else. Others prefer quiet independence. Follow their lead.

Keep sessions short. Ten to fifteen minutes may be ideal. Watch for signs of fatigue or frustration, and gently suggest a break.
Talk about the pictures. If it feels natural, chat about what's being colored "That's a lovely blue bird. Did you ever keep a pet?" Simple conversation can spark pleasant memories.

Celebrate completion. Praise the effort, not just the result. "That looks wonderful!" or "You chose such warm colors!" helps build confidence and joy.

3. The Benefits of Coloring for People with Memory Loss

Coloring offers more than creative fun - it provides gentle cognitive and emotional support.

Relaxation and calm: Focusing on a simple, familiar task helps reduce restlessness and anxiety.

Sense of accomplishment: Completing a page, even partially, builds confidence and satisfaction.

Memory connection: Many designs in this book—flowers, animals, household objects—may awaken pleasant long-term memories, since those memories often remain strong even when recent ones fade.

Focus and coordination: Coloring helps maintain hand–eye coordination and fine motor control in a non-demanding way.

Social interaction: Working side by side encourages companionship and conversation.

Routine and comfort: Familiar activities like coloring can help provide stability in daily life.

The goal is not artistic perfection, but peace, connection, and joy through a simple, soothing activity.

4. Tips for the Best Coloring Experience

Choose the right tools. Thick colored pencils or crayons are easier to hold than thin pencils or markers. Avoid alcohol-based markers, which can bleed through the paper.

Lighting matters. Use bright, even light to reduce eye strain. Natural daylight is ideal.

Encourage comfort. Make sure the table and chair are at a good height, and that the person is sitting comfortably.

Use familiar colors. Bright, high-contrast colors like red, blue, yellow, and green are easiest to recognize.

Display the artwork. Finished pages can be placed in a simple frame or on a bulletin board to build pride and visual joy.

Stay patient. If a page is left unfinished, that's perfectly fine. The experience itself is what matters most.

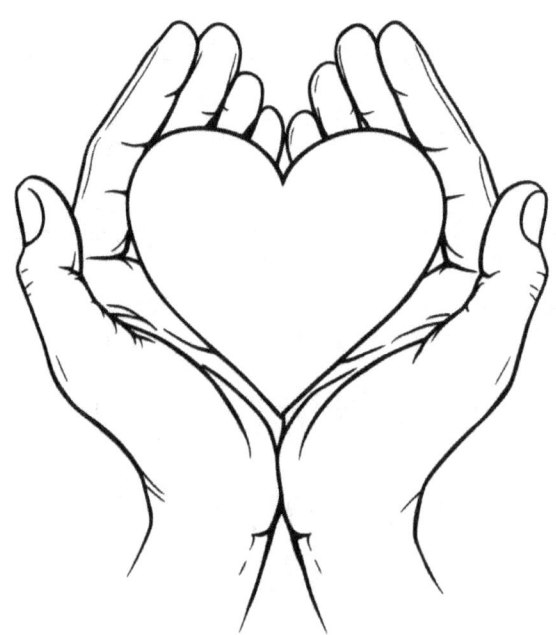

5. About the Author / Our Mission

Nevada Thornton creates books that combine beauty, simplicity, and comfort.

These coloring books are designed with respect for every individual's ability to enjoy art, regardless of age or cognitive challenges. Each page is meant to bring a moment of calm, a spark of recognition, or a smile.

Our mission is to provide families and caregivers with meaningful resources that promote connection, dignity, and happiness—one gentle page at a time.

Thank you for choosing this book to share with someone you care about. May every color bring a little more peace.